D0231863

About the author

Sarah Ockwell-Smith is the mother of four children. She ~~has a~~
BSc in Psychology and worked for several years in Pharmaceutical
Research and Development. Following the birth of her first child,
Sarah retrained as an Antenatal Teacher and Birth and Postnatal
Doula. She has also undertaken training in Hypnotherapy and
Psychotherapy and is a member of the British Sleep Society. Sarah
specialises in gentle parenting methods and is co-founder of the
GentleParenting website www.gentleparentinginternational.com.
She also blogs at www.sarahockwell-smith.com. Sarah is the
author of seven other parenting books: *BabyCalm, ToddlerCalm,*
The Gentle Sleep Book, The Gentle Parenting Book, Why Your
Baby's Sleep Matters, The Gentle Discipline Book and The Gentle
Potty Training Book. She frequently writes for magazines and
newspapers, and is often called upon as a parenting expert for
national television and radio.

HIGHLAND
LIBRARIES

WITHDRAWN

THE GENTLE EATING BOOK

SARAH OCKWELL-SMITH

HIGH LIFE HIGHLAND	
3800 18 0080326 8	
Askews & Holts	16-Jan-2019
613.2083	£14.99

piatkus

PIATKUS

First published in Great Britain in 2018 by Piatkus

1 3 5 7 9 10 8 6 4 2

Copyright © Sarah Ockwell-Smith 2018

The moral right of the author has been asserted.

All rights reserved.
No part of this publication may be reproduced, stored in
a retrieval system, or transmitted in any form or by any means, without
the prior permission in writing of the publisher, nor be otherwise circulated
in any form of binding or cover other than that in which it is published
and without a similar condition including this condition
being imposed on the subsequent purchaser.

Text on pages 38–9 reproduced with
the kind permission of Steven Bratman.

A CIP catalogue record for this book
is available from the British Library.

ISBN 978-0-349-41442-3

Typeset in Stone Serif by M Rules
Printed and bound in Great Britain by
Clays Ltd, St Ives plc

Papers used by Piatkus are from well-managed forests
and other responsible sources.

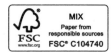

Piatkus
An imprint of
Little, Brown Book Group
Carmelite House
50 Victoria Embankment
London EC4Y 0DZ

An Hachette UK Company
www.hachette.co.uk

www.improvementzone.co.uk

Contents

Acknowledgements

As ever, I am indebted to my family for supporting me while I wrote this book and to all the team at Piatkus and Eve White Literary Agency for making it a reality. I would also like to say a huge thanks to the parents who helped me during the research and writing process, many of whom have allowed me to publish their questions in this book.

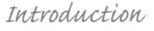

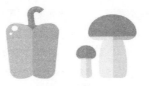

What is Gentle Eating?

W e've all heard the saying, 'You are what you eat'. However, for many parents this could be more accurately phrased as, 'You are what your children eat'. What children do or often don't eat can be a cause of anxiety, shame and constant stress for parents. All too frequently, they pin their self-worth on their children's appetite and weight. Many parents tend to take pride in having raised a 'good eater' and readily accept compliments about their children's table manners, believing that they are the result of good parenting. On the flip side, others worry that they have done something wrong if their baby slips off a weight centile, that their toddler won't eat anything green or when their older child comes home with a letter from school saying that they have an 'unhealthy BMI' and need to lose weight. Judgement from society abounds too.

We are all too quick to blame childhood weight problems on parents, when the issue is far bigger and far more alarming. For such a basic physiological function, eating conjures up so many emotions in parents.

We live in an era of 'information overload' and when this

is combined with such an emotive subject for parents, they simply cannot win. We are bombarded with advice about 'healthy eating', whether from government-sponsored leaflets and parenting magazines or celebrity family cookery books and television slots, featuring expert nutritionists. It is my firm belief, however, that these all do more harm than good, and all the while, stress over eating takes away from the enjoyment of parenting – ironically, often exacerbating the original problem.

Too many books focus on trendy diets and complicated recipes. This book is not one of them. In fact, you won't find a single recipe here. Nor will you find discussions of superfoods, micronutrients or clean eating. This book is different. Instead of providing recipes, nutrition advice, exercise motivation and cookery tips, it will take you on a journey into the physiology and, most importantly, the psychology of eating. Along the way, we will cover many common concerns shared by parents. Topics covered include what to do if your baby is reluctant to eat solids or to take milk from another source when you are breastfeeding but returning to work soon; how to encourage your toddler to eat food that isn't a plain, beige carbohydrate, especially vegetables; what to do if your toddler regresses in their eating, having been an adventurous eater in babyhood; and how to cope when they either don't stop eating, refuse to eat anything or randomly swing between fasting and bingeing. We will also look at eating in school-age children and how to cope with the imposition of school eating rules, weight-based bullying, persistent picky eating and overeating and over-weight. Finally, we will consider teen eating – including and especially dieting and eating disorders – and how to prepare your teen to live independently, while still following healthy, gentle-eating principles.

While I have written this book with several specific, com-monly faced eating issues in mind, it is equally applicable to those reading with no real eating concerns. If you have picked it up to prepare yourself for the journey ahead, rest assured there will be plenty in it for you, no matter how old your child is, or how you have approached eating to date.

To change your child's eating patterns, you must know why they are eating, or perhaps not eating, in a certain way. And I believe it is paramount to understand the basic physiology underpinning appetite, hunger, satiety and taste preferences. Very often, eating behaviours that parents worry about are developmentally normal for the age of their child. Recognising this can take a huge weight off the already heavily burdened shoulders of parents. Therefore, Chapter 1 will take you on a whistle-stop tour of the physiology of eating.

I have written this book to help parents understand not only the way their children eat and to gently nudge them towards more healthy, instinctive eating, but also their own eating patterns and the effect modern society has upon them. It is impossible to separate these issues; they are inextricably intertwined. In fact, understanding the psychology of eating, the silent, unconscious, but perpetual messages we receive about it and the way we ourselves view food and eating is the cornerstone for understanding and changing our children's eating habits. For this reason, Chapter 2 is all about adult eating and our own relationship with food. And it is no coincidence that this chapter appears before any of those explaining eating in children. Put simply, to positively influence the eating habits of your children, you must understand and change your own. Even if you feel that you have a healthy attitude to food, I can guarantee that, sub-consciously, you will have picked up on some erroneous beliefs and unhealthy habits from your own parents, friends, family and other sources.

Parenting forces us to look at ourselves more closely. Our own behaviour and beliefs should always be the starting point for changing those of our children. So although you may be desperate to dive straight into the chapter relevant to your child's age, I would strongly urge you to read chapters 1 and 2 first to gain a far deeper understanding of the theory and tenets of gentle eating. The information in these chapters will help you to understand your own eating and that of your child, to avoid common eating pitfalls, particularly when it comes to the impact of your own behaviour, and to gently steer your child towards a healthier eating pattern, whether you are already facing issues or are reading now in preparation.

In chapters 3 to 7, we will consider eating within smaller age brackets, looking at common eating problems that parents face at each stage of child development. I have divided the book in this way to make it as easy as possible for you to read and, most importantly, make use of. What begins in babyhood often has implications for toddlerhood and beyond. I would therefore urge you, once again, to read as many chapters as possible because they are really all relevant, no matter how old your child is.

My aim in writing this book is to empower you to empower your children. I hope to change your view of eating, to remove a lot of the stress surrounding it and make it into something far less guilt-inducing and far more enjoyable. I hope to help you to raise children who are not only healthy in themselves, but who have a healthy relationship with food – for life. And the way to achieve this, I believe, is to embrace 'gentle eating'.

What is gentle eating?

Throughout this book – and indeed, in its title – I use the term 'gentle eating' to sum up a healthy and relaxed ethos about eating. Gentle eating encompasses four main beliefs that apply in any situation and at any age:

1. Gentle eating is mindful

Being mindful of our eating requires us to focus on the whole experience. That means we are not distracted when we eat and that we do not eat as a distraction. We eat when we are hungry, being aware of the signals our bodies are sending us, and we stop eating when we are full. We don't eat to silence uncomfortable emotions and we are aware of any beliefs or conditioning from our own upbringing that may cause us subconsciously to repeat patterns of eating.

From a parenting perspective, eating mindfully means dissociating food from not only your own emotions but also your child's. It means not using food as a reward for 'being good' or as a distraction to keep your child calm or quiet. And it means not labelling food as 'good' or 'bad' and being aware of how your own beliefs about eating can influence your children. Being mindful also means avoiding distractions at mealtimes, whether that's eating in front of the television or having intense conversations over the dinner table about something your child has or hasn't done at school. It also involves being aware of your own feelings around your child's eating and not taking their behaviour personally or extrapolating it as a judgement of your parenting skills.

2. Gentle eating is empowering

Following gentle-eating principles empowers all members of the family: parents are empowered to trust their children and their own parenting skills, based on a sound understanding and knowledge of normal, healthy eating; and children are empowered to follow their body's own signals and self-regulate their food intake, rather than rely on instructions from their parents or messages from society. This will have far-reaching effects (including the possibility of empowering their own children in the future) and creates a positive spiral, enabling everyone in the family to feel more secure and confident.

3. Gentle eating is respectful

When parents understand the psychological and physiological effects and roles of eating, they can show true respect for their children. Far too many parents believe they are doing 'the best thing' for their children by force-feeding them, rewarding, praising, chastising and restricting their food intake. This erroneous belief unfortunately serves to disrespect children by misunderstanding them.

The informed beliefs of gentle eating allow parents to afford their children the respect that they deserve. This, in turn, teaches children to respect their bodies and the marvellous things that they achieve every day, which can only be positive for their overall well-being and self-esteem.

4. Gentle eating is authoritative

When it comes to childhood eating, most commonly parents fall into two camps.

On the one hand, there are the authoritarians, who seek to control what their children eat. They restrict foods, often banning what they believe to be unhealthy, or 'bad' food. Portion sizes are prescribed – not too much and not too little – plate clearing is often enforced and rewarded, eating is done on a schedule, with routine mealtimes and consequences if the children don't eat 'well'. Personal preferences and dislikes are not truly respected if they are believed to be 'unhealthy'.

On the other hand, there are the permissives – those who give their children full control, with little attempt to regulate any aspect of eating, particularly when it comes to choice of foods offered. Permissives may give up trying to offer healthy food or abandon all hope of any table manners. Permissive eating tends not to be mindful and distractions often abound – for instance, eating while watching television to encourage the child to eat more.

In the middle of these two styles is authoritative parenting. Authoritatives strike a balance between too much control and too little. They are informed and understand both the physiology and psychology of eating. They respect their children and seek to empower them through their eating by taking most of the control of some of the more mature aspects, such as choosing and preparing foods and deciding when to seek professional help. They don't attach emotions to eating, don't reward or punish; instead, they encourage the development of self-regulation.

Gentle eating is very much in line with authoritative parenting and, in my opinion, it is the only approach that is mindful of the child's eating today, while also being concerned with their relationship with food in the years to come. Gentle eating can help not only to change our children's well-being for the better, but our own as parents, too. It is sensible, intuitive and, most importantly, supported by a growing body of scientific evidence, which I will refer to throughout the book.

Gentle-eating principles apply at any age, from the day your baby is born to the day your teenager leaves for college and beyond. In fact, you may find that a lot of information in this book is helpful to you too, as an adult. However, it is not a quick fix. It is a lifestyle ethos and requires a shift not only in the way you feed your child, but also in how you yourself think about food.

To change children's eating for the better, we must first start with understanding what normal eating looks like and the physiological processes that govern it. Sometimes that means re-educating ourselves, in order to change the way our children eat. And a wonderful and unexpected side effect of this is that often this knowledge can bring a new sense of freedom to our own relationship with food.

PLEASE NOTE

The information contained here is not a replacement for medical advice. I have written this book presuming that your child is otherwise healthy, emotionally and physically. It does not cover medical or pathological extremes of eating, nor does it deal with specific psychological or physiological disorders. If you feel that your child's eating may require special attention, please listen to your instinct and seek professional medical advice from a qualified doctor.

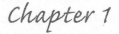

Chapter 1

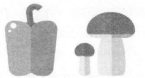

The Physiology of Eating

sn't it ironic that so many books, articles, television programmes and websites discussing 'healthy eating' for children focus only on how to change eating, without helping parents to appreciate what normal eating looks like in the first place? If we don't know how hunger and appetite work, why taste preferences exist and how our lives impact on them, how are we ever going to truly understand how to gently change the way our children eat?

If you are reading this book as preparation, having not yet experienced any problems, this chapter will help you to gently steer your child's eating on a positive course for the years to come. If you have a pre-existing worry or concern over your child's eating, then it will help you to uncover some of the root causes, and to resolve the issue as gently and positively as possible.

In my opinion, jumping straight into tempting healthy recipes is both naive and unhelpful. A basic introduction to the physiology of the eating process is needed first because knowing how things work must always be the starting point. In this chapter I will begin by looking at some of the most important language around eating, namely hunger, appetite, satiation and satiety, comparing and contrasting these terms, while taking a brief look at the physiology underpinning each of them. Next, I will look at certain influences upon our eating, especially sleep and stress. Following this, I will cover the physiology of taste and, importantly, taste preferences and cravings – a concept that we will return to throughout the book. This combined knowledge will provide a firm foundation from which to consider eating patterns at each age, from birth through to adulthood, as covered in later chapters.

This chapter constitutes important foundation learning, whether you have a newborn on a 'milk-only' diet, are struggling with a toddler who is reluctant to eat meals you have slaved over for hours or are looking to avoid the perils of a dieting teenager.

The physiology of hunger and satiety

Confusingly, when discussing hunger and its presence or absence, society often mixes up different terminology and concepts. To understand the physiology of hunger and satiety (the sensation of *not* being hungry), we must first differentiate them from other similar sensations, namely appetite and satiation. This is vital when considering gentle eating because we cannot be mindful about something we do not truly comprehend. So let's begin with a brief look at the terminology.

- **Appetite** is the word used to describe the response to a blend of psychological and physiological stimuli (such as smell, thought, memory and preferences), which can lead the individual to begin or delay eating. Hunger need not be present for appetite to be heightened.

- **Hunger** is used to describe the intrinsic, uncomfortable physiological sensation caused by a lack of food, which leads the individual to seek it. Appetite is of less importance when true hunger is experienced.

- **Satiation** relates to the amount eaten during a meal. It describes the physiological and psychological responses experienced at the time of consuming food, resulting in sensations of fullness and satisfaction (again, both physiological and psychological), leading the individual to stop eating.

- **Satiety** relates to the space between meals. It is about the level of fullness and satisfaction experienced by an individual after they have eaten, resulting in the inhibition of further eating for an amount of time, until hunger returns. While satiety is guided predominantly by physiological processes, psychological ones undoubtedly play a role too.

How hunger occurs

Hunger represents the body's physiological need to consume more food. This need should be differentiated from wanting food. Hunger keeps us alive and our bodies functioning. It does not involve psychological preferences or desires. The most common symptom of hunger is a feeling of emptiness in the stomach, often accompanied by muscular contractions (or hunger pangs) and sometimes a 'growling' or rumbling noise in the stomach. These symptoms originate in the stomach, which sends electrical signals via the vagus nerve to the brain. This effect is largely triggered by the secretion of the hormone ghrelin, and by metabolic signals such as the secretion of the hormone insulin, which results in a drop in the body's blood glucose levels.

How satiation and satiety occur

Satiation occurs when we have eaten enough food. Due to a delay between the swallowing and digesting of food, the body needs a short-term signal to indicate that it is time to stop consuming food, to prevent overeating. Research indicates that this 'quick-fix' signal occurs as a mix of psychological, mechanical and chemical factors.[1] Psychological factors include something known as sensory-specific satiety, a term used to describe the decrease in satisfaction from eating more of the same substance and thus a decrease in appetite due to the novelty of the taste wearing off. Mechanical factors include gastric distension (stretching of the stomach), which causes a sensation of fullness. Chemical factors include the taste and smell of food. This three-pronged effect helps us to feel full and, importantly, to cease eating before digestion of the meal is advanced. The state of satiety is achieved when certain levels of insulin, amino acids and glucose are detected in the blood and by the oxidation of nutrients in the liver. When the level of these chemicals decreases, satiety does so too and, ultimately, hunger returns.[2] Once again, satiety is largely hormonally regulated. The hormone cholecystokinin, which is produced when the gall bladder contracts, inhibits feelings of hunger. Perhaps the most important hormone related to satiety and inhibition of hunger, however, is leptin. This is produced by fat cells in the body; therefore, theoretically, the more fat stores in the body, the more leptin is released and the stronger the messages reaching the brain, causing inhibition of hunger and the further accumulation of excess fat stores.

Sensory-specific satiety

Sensory-specific satiety results in a decrease in satisfaction when eating more of the same substance. The lack of novelty in the taste of the food being eaten leads to a decrease in appetite for that specific foodstuff. One study showed this phenomenon in practice, when researchers asked adults to consume a glass of chocolate milk.[3] After consuming the drink, they were asked to play a game whereby they could obtain either crisps or chocolate milk. Half were offered more chocolate milk and half some crisps. Those who were playing for more chocolate milk displayed a decreased liking of the taste and smell of chocolate milk and less motivation to obtain more, when compared to the motivation and preferences of the group playing for crisps. Sensory-specific satiety in humans reflects a decrease in both food liking and food wanting and illustrates our preference for varied foods. This concept shows us the impact the sensory experience of eating can have – both positive and negative – on our appetites. Sensory-specific satiety also helps us to understand one way in which our thoughts, preferences and sensory experience of a food can limit our hunger in the absence of true physiological satiety.

THE HORMONES OF HUNGER AND SATIETY

As mentioned previously, hunger and satiety are governed by chemical signals and their impact on the body. The following table shows the basic effect on hunger levels of the most important eating-related hormones. →

Hormone	Action	Effect on hunger
Ghrelin	Sends messages to the brain to stimulate hunger and prepares the gastrointestinal tract for incoming food by increasing motility and gastric acid secretion.	Stimulates
Leptin	Signals to the brain that the body has enough stores of fat.	Inhibits
Insulin	Increasing levels of insulin causes a drop in the body's glucose levels.	Stimulates
Cholecystokinin	Decreases the rate of digestion.	Inhibits

DIFFERENTIATING APPETITE FROM HUNGER

The following table provides a brief overview of the differences between appetite and hunger and how an individual may respond to the sensations they arouse.

Appetite	Hunger
Largely psychological process	Largely physiological process
Sudden onset, can be ignored if preoccupied with another activity	Gradual onset that slowly becomes more urgent
Desire for specific foods	Desire to eat often overrides food choice
Sensations are more 'in the mind' and described as a yearning, longing or craving	Accompanied by physical sensations, such as a 'growling tummy' and hunger pangs

Appetite	Hunger
Desire to eat is often not diminished once food has been consumed	Desire to eat again disappears for several hours after consuming food
Continuation of eating after a feeling of fullness because of enjoyment	Eating ceases once full
Emotions and food are strongly linked to each other	No emotions involved

The most important message to take away when differentiating between hunger and appetite is that hunger is a physiological need and appetite is an emotional want. While the two may occur together, they are very different, and understanding this is paramount when it comes to parents considering their children's eating habits. Gentle eating focuses on being mindful or, put another way, eating for hunger. When we link emotions and eating, be that through rewarding, bribing, threatening or shaming, we completely misunderstand how appetite and hunger work. Gentle eating must be free of emotion as much as possible, for both parent and child, in a way that also affords respect for the child's individual eating preferences or appetite.

The psychology of appetite

While hunger, satiation and satiety are predominantly physiological, appetite, in contrast, has a large psychological component. Appetite can really be summarised as food wants and, very often, these can overshadow food needs. (If eating was based on need only, the world would not be experiencing such a rising obesity problem.) The psychological processes that distinguish appetite from hunger are one of the keys for parents who wish to move towards a more gentle, mindful and respectful view of their children's eating.

Appetite encompasses a broad array of variables, such as:

- individual taste preferences

- sensory likes and dislikes

- temperature preferences (preferring to eat food hot, cold, or lukewarm)

- visual appeal

- aroma

- the amount of same food consumed

- memories and emotions linked to previous experiences of specific foods

- the social aspect (for instance, sharing food with friends)

- learned behaviour surrounding food (for instance, the idea that certain food should be eaten at specific times of the day)

- learned beliefs about food (that certain food is 'good' or 'bad', for example).

These thought processes can and do overshadow hunger, affecting whether we choose to eat when we are not hungry – or not eat when we are.

The hunger–satiety cycle – a summary

Before we consider how aspects of our modern-day lives impact on our physiology and the regulation of eating, I thought it would be a good idea to sum up what we have covered so far in this chapter. The following diagram shows the cycle of hunger, satiation and satiety and the different hormonal changes involved at each point. Remember, hunger is not the same as appetite, although appetite plays a role in the seeking, choice of and continuation or cessation of eating food.

THE HUNGER-SATIETY CYCLE

HUNGER
* Emptiness of stomach detected along with lowered levels of nutrients in the intestines
* Gastric cramping occurs, known commonly as 'hunger pangs'
* Hormone ghrelin released

SEEK FOOD, BEGIN EATING
* Sensory influences on choice of food – including the smell, taste and sight of certain foods
* Thought processes and memories affect our choices

CONTINUE EATING
* Cognitive influences on the amount we eat include eating in the presence of others, the time of day, our relationship with food and our liking of certain foods

SATIATION, CEASE EATING
* Sensory specific satiety
* Stretch receptors in gut sense fullness
* Nutrients detected in intestines

SATIETY
* Glucose, amino acids and insulin levels in blood reduce hunger
* Feeling of 'fullness' remains
* Ghrelin levels decrease
* Leptin inhibits feelings of hunger

The physiology of taste

The sense of taste, or gustation to give it its official name, helps to drive our appetite and enables us to stay safe by protecting us from poisonous foodstuffs. We innately prefer savoury, salty and sweet tastes, over bitter and sour ones, most likely because the latter two are more commonly found in foods that are toxic to us. Our sense of taste develops over time, however, due to a blend of repeated exposure and maturing cognitive abilities, when we learn that not all bitter and sour tastes are a threat to our survival. This idea is one I will examine in much more detail in Chapter 5, when we look at toddler and preschooler eating.

Our sense of taste occurs in taste receptor cells, 50–150 of which are contained in our individual taste buds. Our taste receptor cells send messages about the sensation of taste to the brainstem, which, in turn, controls whether we continue or stop eating a particular foodstuff, as well as triggering a chain of events to aid digestion, such as an increase in salivation. Most of our taste buds are found in small bumps on the surface of the tongue, called papillae, and while the tongue's papillae are visible to the naked eye, taste buds are not. While previously it was believed that different areas of the tongue are responsible for different tastes, these 'maps' have now been shown to be inaccurate, with taste buds not having such clear boundaries.

The sensation of taste is an individual experience: some people will respond more strongly to certain tastes, while others simply seem to taste more strongly. This genetic difference is, in part, due to the number of papillae and taste buds found on the tongue, with more being found in those who experience stronger taste sensations. Around a quarter of the population are known as 'supertasters', the supertaster gene appearing to amplify the taste of food, especially bitter tastes.

There are five known specific tastes experienced by humans:

- **Bitter** Examples include coffee and high-cocoa-content dark chocolate. Bitter tastes also commonly occur in plants or animals that are toxic.

- **Salty** Examples include food in brine. Salty tastes allow the body to regulate the balance of electrolytes.

- **Sour** Examples include lemons, limes and vinegar. Sourness allows the body to detect acid levels in foods.

- **Sweet** Examples include honey and fruits. Sweetness usually indicates foods rich in energy content.

- **Umami** Examples include cheese, meat and foods containing monosodium glutamate. Umami usually indicates the presence of amino acids.

The sense of taste is also impacted by the sense of smell and it is the combination of 'events' in the mouth, nose and brain that gives us the flavour of a food.

Contrary to popular belief, strong cravings for a specific taste or food are rooted firmly in psychology and not physiology and do not indicate a deficiency of a certain nutrient. Rather, cravings occur because of our experiences, emotions and memories surrounding food. This is an idea we will return to again in Chapter 2 (see page 23).

The effect of sleep on hunger and appetite

Eating and sleep have a strong relationship: what we eat can affect our sleep and our sleep, in turn, can affect what we eat.

Foods that are rich in the amino acid tryptophan aid the onset of sleep. Tryptophan is one of the building blocks of serotonin, a neurotransmitter that helps to modulate the sleep/wake cycle in the brain, as well as regulating emotional stability. Imbalances in serotonin levels can, therefore, result in disrupted circadian rhythms (otherwise known as body clocks), as well as a lack of emotional stability. Tryptophan is commonly found in eggs, poultry, whole wheat and nuts. Food can inhibit sleep too, the most common culprit being caffeine, which acts a stimulant and sleep suppressor.

Earlier in this chapter we considered the effect of the hormones ghrelin and leptin on hunger and satiety. (Ghrelin stimulates hunger, while leptin inhibits it.) Ordinarily, when we sleep leptin levels increase, which helps us to stay asleep for several hours, without waking as a result of hunger. Less sleep, however, means less leptin is secreted and higher levels of ghrelin circulate in the body, stimulating hunger. If sleep deprivation continues, leptin levels will remain low, while ghrelin levels rise.[4] This imbalance causes an increase in hunger, despite the body not needing fuel, which can lead to weight gain or difficulty in losing excess weight. Research shows an increased risk of obesity in both children and adults with consistently short sleep periods.[5] This concept is of great importance when thinking about teenagers, who tend to get less sleep at night towards the end of primary school or the start of secondary school. This sleep reduction is in part due to a change in their circadian rhythms and a shift towards later sleep onset – a pattern that is clearly at odds with school start times. We cannot, however, discount the impact of screens and their use by older children at night. Coupled with the shift in body clocks, this can give us a potential explanation for rising levels of obesity in adolescence. This idea, and how to tackle it, is examined in some depth in Chapter 7 (see page 187).

The effect of stress on hunger and appetite

Like sleep deprivation, stress can have a similar hunger-stimulating effect on the body. Admittedly, short-term stress has a limited inhibitory effect on hunger, thanks to the 'fight-or-flight' response, which causes us not to want to eat if we are anxious or nervous about something. Chronic, long-lasting stress, on the other hand, can drive the body to eat more due to the secretion of the stress hormone cortisol. Usually, cortisol levels fall back to normal at the end of a stressful event. However, in some cases the stressor may remain and so too the stress response, which, in turn, can cause the hormone ghrelin to be elevated, triggering hunger. Research has also found that the high ghrelin levels that accompany stress may help us to cope with any resulting anxiety and depression.[6]

Cortisol can also cause individuals, particularly females, to crave high-fat and high-sugar foods.[7] This effect may have a small physiological component, as well as the more common psychological one. High-fat and high-sugar foods can have a slight 'numbing' effect on the part of the brain that is responsible for producing stress and anxiety.[8] Stress-related eating also has a strong psychological component, with learned reactions, memories and conditioned responses. If a person learns that cake is used to palliate stress in childhood, the chances are they will continue to eat cake when stressed in adulthood, even if the cake has no physiological effects on their body's stress response. This is an important point that we will return to in Chapter 2.

These new insights into the physiology and psychology of eating mean it is necessary to take a much more holistic approach. Eating encompasses many variables and these must be understood if we want to make a positive change to our children's relationship with food, or start them off on the most positive path. It is not as simple as previous generations have made out. New understandings in science mean that we must move on from the outdated behaviourist approaches to eating that hinge on praise, reward and consequences – those that involve giving a sticker if a child nibbles on a Brussels sprout, or sending them to bed hungry if they turn their nose up at dinner. Everything is interlinked: biology, emotions and sleep.

We must also consider eating from an evolutionary perspective – while science moves on quickly, evolution does so much more slowly. What, if any, eating practices (especially those exhibited by children) may hark back to a different era? Are these evolutionary kickbacks wrong, just because they don't fit into our modern-day view of eating? This is a question that we will come back to throughout the following chapters, particularly in Chapter 5, when we look at eating in one- to four-year-olds.

To close this chapter, I would like to remind you of the four basic tenets of gentle eating. It is: mindful, empowering, respectful and authoritative. We have seen how appetite, hunger, satiation and satiety are governed by psychological and physiological components, which is why the mindful aspect of gentle eating is so important. In order to help our children to eat mindfully, we should empower them to trust their own bodily cues, via an authoritative and respectful parenting style. These last three tenets of gentle eating are all interwoven and interdependent and each is as important as the other. We must understand the full spectrum of eating influences to fulfil these gentle-eating goals with our children.

We've looked at some of the physiological influences at play with your child's eating. In Chapter 2, we will look at some of the psychological influences that affect how, what and when children eat, starting with the biggest psychological influence of all – you!

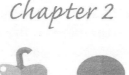

Chapter 2

They Are What We Eat – Adult Eating and Why It Matters

You may be wondering why this book includes a chapter on adult eating, when you are concerned about your child's, not your own. You may also be tempted to skip this chapter and go straight to the one appropriate for your child's age. There is, however, a very good reason why it is not only included in this book, but also appears before those concerned with children's eating – because if we want to improve the latter, we must make sure that we, as adults, are setting a good example. Sadly, most of us do anything but.

Many of the worries we have about our children's eating are rooted in our own disordered eating and dysfunctional beliefs. If our aim is to help our children to follow a gentle-eating ethos – one that is mindful, empowering, respectful and authoritative – we must follow the same rules ourselves. Before we can even begin to tackle any eating-related concerns with our children, we must work with our own, otherwise we will pass them on or create new problems based on them in our children. We may even learn that what we believed to be their issues are in fact our own and they are eating entirely normally. This is why this chapter is included and why it comes before the others. Please do take the time to read it.

Your relationship with food

How do you feel about your eating? Do you feel that it is under control? Do you feel relaxed around food? Are you happy with your body? Do you feel that your relationship with food is healthy? Or do you feel that there are elements of eating that you struggle with as an adult? How would you feel if your child grew up with the same thoughts and feelings about their body and eating as you? If any of these questions leave you feeling a little uncomfortable, then it is especially important for you to read this chapter, in order that you can try to avoid passing on any of your own unhealthy beliefs to your child. If, however, you feel that you have a good relationship with eating and with your body, then this chapter may serve to highlight why this is and how you can pass on your own positive thoughts to your children, avoiding common pitfalls that may appear over the next few years. Either way, this must be your starting point, whether you are coming from a position of reading in preparation, without any specific worries or concerns, or you are looking for solutions to specific problems that you have with your child's eating.

Hangovers from childhood

Many of our beliefs and behaviours surrounding eating stem from our own childhoods. Often, they are a conditioned response to something that happened decades ago. Eating and food are commonly intertwined with our childhood memories – both good and bad. As parents, as much as we think we may be, or indeed hope to be, we are not objective about food and eating. And we may subconsciously influence our children and their eating as a result.

While we can't change what happened to us, we can recognise its impact and be mindful of it, so as not to repeat the cycle again and again. Think back to food in your own childhood and the roles of your parents, grandparents, school-dinner ladies or other adults. Collectively, I call these individuals 'the Food Police'; I suspect you had quite a few of them in your life when you were growing up. Do you remember hearing them say any of the following?

- 'Good girl, you ate all your dinner.'

- 'Well done, what a lovely clean plate.'

- 'Come on, eat up – there are children starving in Africa.'

- 'Just one bite – it won't kill you.'

- 'Eat your crusts up – they make your hair curl.'

- 'If you don't eat your carrots, you won't be able to see in the dark.'

- 'No pudding for you if you don't eat up your dinner.'

- 'Don't eat that now, you'll spoil your appetite.'

- 'Just one more mouthful, then you can have some ice cream.'

- 'You're such a good girl; you've got such a healthy appetite.'

- 'You're not getting down from this table unless you finish your food.'

- 'If you don't eat it, then you'll go straight to your room and be hungry.'

- 'If you eat that, your teeth will rot and fall out.'

- 'If you don't finish your meal, you won't get a treat.'

- 'Eat up quickly, otherwise your brother will eat it for you.'

- 'Cheer up, stop crying – here's a nice chocolate bar to help you feel better.'

Some of these statements may bring up uncomfortable memories of your childhood, and may even begin to remind you of how some of your own eating behaviours have been formed. Becoming mindful of the subconscious drivers of your own eating behaviour is a significant stepping stone towards following and achieving gentle-eating principles. But even if none of these statements rings a bell for you, being aware of the impact of your own words and those of any other adults who care for your child is important in order to help prevent any emotional eating issues from developing. Awareness – being mindful – is always an incredibly important first step towards adopting a gentle-eating mindset.

I was a 'good girl' when I was a child. I ate a lot of food, wasn't especially picky about what I ate, cleared my plate and rarely let anything go to waste – and I was regularly praised for it. My self-esteem was quite strongly tied to being 'a good eater'. I felt proud of my eating and eating, as a result, made me feel good. Can you tell where this is going? Fast-forward thirty years or so and I struggle with regulating my eating. I eat to make myself feel better when I'm sad or stressed, just as I was encouraged to do as a child. Eating is how I make myself feel good. It has also taken me many years to overcome the guilt of leaving food on my plate, especially a substantial amount. I finally resolved the wastage issue by getting chickens, which eat pretty much any food that is left over in our house. I still feel pangs of guilt if I must discard food when we're away from home though. The emotional eating has taken much longer and much more work on my behalf to undo. I know where my food issues stem from, but they are so hard to overcome.

Once you understand why you behave the way you do around food, you can then begin to change the deeply ingrained patterns. But what if you don't, or can't, change them? Well, you risk passing them on to your own children and, in turn, any future grandchildren and so on.

Emotional eating and the link with reward

Do you ever eat out of sadness, anxiety or boredom? The British often say that 'a good cup of tea' helps solve everything; for many, however, that cup of tea is accompanied by a couple of biscuits, a bar of chocolate or a slice of cake. It is no surprise, then, that so many of us turn to sugary treats to console ourselves, because we were placated by them in childhood. Food can be a quick, easy and superficially successful way for parents to keep a lid on children's emotions. Sweets and chocolate are often used to quieten and distract toddlers about to tantrum, children who have fallen and hurt themselves, and even teenagers who are upset about falling out with a friend. But what happens over the years when that child learns to rely on eating to achieve an emotional status quo? Eating stops being mindful; it is no longer solely a response to hunger, physical satiety is overridden by a lack of emotional satiety and disordered eating becomes a way of life.

Research has shown that children are drawn to high-fat and sugary foods when their parents use food to regulate their emotions or as a reward for certain behaviour.[1] While the link between regulating children's emotions with foods and the development of emotional eating may be fairly obvious, many parents aren't aware of the connection between using food as a reward and emotional eating. The basics of both, however, are the same. Using food to help children feel good, whether that is a lollipop given to stop them crying after a fall or a chocolate bar given as a reward for a job well done, creates a relationship for them between eating and feelings. Put simply, if children are used to associating food with feeling good or feeling better, it is no surprise that as they grow up they eat when they are experiencing uncomfortable emotions. And the food chosen to override sadness, anxiety or stress will always be one that is associated with being a 'treat', or reward. Scientists are clear that using food as a reward in childhood increases the risk of disordered and emotional eating as the child grows.[2]

It isn't only children, however, who are rewarded with food; adults often are too. Can you remember a time when you have been to a restaurant or food shop with your children in tow and have declared that you were going to treat yourself, perhaps for being 'good'? These are the sorts of behaviours and self-talk that children pick up on. If they see you using food as a treat for yourself, even if you don't use it to treat them, they may still develop a form of emotional eating.

Unfortunately, rewarding with food or using it to regulate emotions is rife in our society, for both children and adults. One of the keys for preventing emotional eating developing in childhood is to understand it and stop it.

Giving food a personality – the problem with labelling

Many adults tend to anthropomorphise food or ascribe human traits to it. The classic here is calling food 'good' or 'naughty'. These and other similar labels don't belong to food, however – they are figments of our imaginations and a projection of our conditioned, disordered beliefs surrounding eating. The same is true of the words 'healthy' and 'unhealthy'. These terms should be used to describe the whole of a person's diet and attitude to food, not specific parts of them. Cake is not unhealthy, vegetables are not healthy; it is the amount of them that we eat, how often we eat them and in what combination that is.

There is an interesting psychological effect caused by our beliefs and labelling of so-called 'healthy' foods, known as 'the health halo effect'. This occurs when we believe that a food which may have some healthy aspects is completely virtuous. For instance, we may believe that something labelled organic is healthier than it is because of the organic label. Research conducted in Germany looking at the impact of labelling on behaviour found that foods with 'healthy' labels had a very different impact on people who were trying to lose weight.[3] Researchers found that the study participants ate significantly more trail mix when it carried the label 'fitness snack', rather than just 'trail mix'. In addition, when participants were given the opportunity to use an exercise bike, those who had eaten the trail mix with the 'fitness' label exercised less than those who had consumed the same food labelled just 'trail mix', somehow believing that they needed to exercise less if they had eaten a food intended for 'fitness', even though they had consumed more.

Why does this matter, you may ask. It matters because the

way in which we, as adults, label and anthropomorphise food has a direct influence on how our children view it and, by extension, on how and what they eat. Research into the eating habits of four- and five-year-olds has found that children are less likely to eat something if it carries an outcome-based label indicating that it is good for them in some way (whether literally, i.e. on the packaging, or via caregivers) – for instance, if they are told a certain food 'makes you strong' or 'helps you to read'.[4] The research also found that if a food is labelled as being good for them, children believe that it must therefore be less tasty.

This sort of labelling doesn't just affect our psychology though. Unbelievably, it can also affect our physiological response to food. Researchers from Yale University in the USA conducted an experiment with a group of forty-six adult volunteers.[5] The participants were asked to attend two sessions at a hospital research unit, a week apart, to help test some new milkshakes that were being developed, with different nutrient contents. On both visits they were given an identical milkshake containing 380 calories, although they were told they were different. On one visit, they were informed that the milkshake was a high-fat, high-calorie 'indulgent' one, containing 620 calories, and on the other they were told that they were being given a low-fat, low-calorie 'sensible' milkshake containing 140 calories. Half of the participants received the 'sensible' milkshake first, while half received the 'indulgent' milkshake first. In both cases, participants were asked to consume the milkshake in its entirety within ten minutes. Once they had done so, researchers measured their ghrelin levels (the hunger hormone) at three different points in time. What they found was astounding. Those who had consumed the 'indulgent' milkshake showed steep declines in ghrelin levels and said that they felt fuller for longer. Those who had consumed the 'sensible' milkshake had a much smaller drop in ghrelin levels and reported feeling less full. The results of this experiment prove the amazing power of mindset and belief when it comes to our eating behaviour.

There is one last way in which adults use food-related labelling and this is perhaps the most concerning of all. Calling children 'cupcake', 'sweetie pie', 'treacle' and the like indicates to them that sweet foods are the ones to aspire to. None of us calls our children 'little cauliflower' or 'beef casserole'. What effect does this have on our children's preferences? There is a strong chance that they will favour those foods we use to positively identify them. If we want our children to have a healthy relationship with food, it makes sense not to use foodstuffs as terms of endearment.

Avoiding food 'labels' and being mindful (one of the four basic tenets of gentle eating) around food means we, and our children, can take more control over the eating experience. Respect, another important tenet of gentle eating, allows our children to have individual choice and preferences, rather than us unwittingly passing on our own tastes or inhibiting or encouraging eating, via labelling. This labelling is often deeply ingrained in us, usually stemming back to our own childhoods. It takes time to undo, but being aware – or mindful – of it is a great starting point.

The social niceties and norms of eating

Whenever I'm running a question-and-answer session with parents I'm almost always asked the following questions:

'How do I get my child to eat dinner? She just won't eat in the evening.'

'How do I get my child to eat his main meal before his dessert?'

'My daughter will only eat cornflakes for dinner. How do I get her to eat what we're eating?'

In each of these scenarios I ask the parents to consider what exactly their problem is and most importantly, who has that problem. After some discussion, the answers always come down to adult expectations. As adults, much of our eating is uninstinctive: we eat according to the clock, not our hunger, and we eat to socially prescribed 'rules', not to our appetite. The real problem comes when we expect our children to follow our own unnatural eating practices. Take, for example, choice of foods. Who decided that cornflakes should only be eaten first thing in the morning? Why can't they be eaten in the afternoon or evening? What makes them a suitable breakfast food, yet an unsuitable offering for lunch or dinner? What would happen if you ate a sandwich in the morning and cornflakes for lunch? The answer is obviously, nothing. So why are we so fixated on 'breakfast food', 'lunch food' and 'dinner food'? The same goes for a main meal and dessert. Why can't dessert come first? Or at the same time as the main meal? Certainly, if it did, we would lose the labelling of the main meal being 'healthy' and something that must be eaten before the 'unhealthy' dessert.

Another unwritten rule is about when we eat and how much is eaten at what time. As adults, we tend to eat three times a day – breakfast, lunch and dinner – with perhaps one or two small snacks in between. Our evening meal is almost always the biggest meal of the day, aside from on Sunday, perhaps, when it is common to eat the main meal of the day at lunchtime. Usual times to eat are 7 a.m., between 12 and 2 p.m., and anywhere between 5 and 8 p.m. This pattern of eating, however, is not mindful. Nor is it particularly instinctive. As adults, we have learned to ignore our hunger and satiety signals and to eat instead at prescribed times. We eat if we're not hungry if it is a mealtime, we don't eat when we are hungry if it is not a mealtime and we save most of our eating for the evening. When children come along and they want to eat their lunch at 10 a.m., followed by a huge meal at 2 p.m. and then nothing else until the next morning, we think their eating is problematic. We stress over them not eating dinner or eating too much in the morning. The sad reality is, however, that *we* are the abnormal eaters, not our children, who eat when they are hungry – regardless of when that is – and stop when they are full, even if that satiety clashes with a mealtime. We, as adults, override the signals our bodies are giving us, eating by the clock and long-held, undisputed, social rules. Perhaps we could learn something from the more mindful and instinctive eating of our children, rather than trying to shape them to fit our own, non-mindful eating patterns.

Adult body image and mirroring negative self-talk

Our own body image has a powerful impact on our eating behaviours. In Chapter 1, we learned how stress affects eating (see page 21). Persistent feelings of a lack of self-worth or body hatred often result in uncomfortable, stressful feelings. This stress can cause us either to overeat or to restrict our eating in a quest to lose weight and feel better about ourselves. Either way, a negative body image and disordered eating often go hand in hand.

How you feel about your own body matters hugely to your children. They are not exempt from the impact of body image, which can – and does – have as much impact on them as it does on us. If you talk about being fat, wanting to lose weight, your 'gross', wobbly tummy and big bottom, or your ugly stretch marks in front of your children, you demonstrate to them how to judge their own bodies. If you, as an adult, are hypercritical of your appearance, you teach them to behave in the same way towards their own bodies. Research has shown that parental body image, particularly the mother's, has an impact on that of children as young as four and remains a strong influencer throughout adolescence, especially for girls.[6] If you want your child to be happy in his or her own skin and appreciative of what they have, then you must start learning to accept your own body – a tough call in a world full of celebrity culture, cosmetic surgery, Botox, social media and photoshopped images.

To help our children grow up with self-esteem, independent of their looks, we first need to break free of the trend ourselves. Changing our language is a good starting point. The British actress Kate Winslet was once asked in an interview about body image and how she influences her daughter, Mia. She replied: 'As a child, I never heard one woman say to me, "I love my body". Not my mother, my older sister, my best friend. No one woman has ever said, "I am proud of my body". So, I make sure to say it to Mia, because a positive physical outlook has to start at an early age.' Modelling a positive image through language may seem slightly odd and uncomfortable at first, but the more you do it, the easier it becomes. Consider some of the following common phrases and what we might replace them with to make them more positive:

Negative body talk	Positive body talk
My belly is so fat and wobbly	I'm so grateful for my belly, for helping to nourish me
My thighs are so big	I love my strong thighs; they carry me every day
My bottom is huge	I really appreciate my bottom; the padding makes it comfortable when I sit down
My arms are too long	I love my long and graceful arms; they help me to dance

Negative body talk	Positive body talk
I hate my stretch marks	Every mark reminds me of when you were in my tummy. I'm so happy to have a memory of that special time
I wish I didn't have so many wrinkles	The lines on my face remind me of all the learning I have done in my life, and how much wiser I am now

Next time you catch yourself about to say something negative about your body, especially if your children are nearby, try to think about how you can reframe your thoughts into something complimentary and positive.

Diet culture and the dangers of perceived deprivation

Estimates suggest that two thirds of all adults in the UK are on a diet 'most of the time'. This alone should tell us everything we need to know about dieting – that it doesn't work.[7]

The diet industry is worth billions of pounds, and it thrives on insecurity and failure – our insecurity about our own bodies, perpetuated by the images it uses of slim and toned young adults and our repeated 'failure' to lose the weight and keep it off. Science has shown time and again that diets don't work. If anything, they make us gain weight, not lose it. Research has found that people may lose around 5–10 per cent of their body weight when they begin dieting, but most go on to regain all they lost and usually a bit more.[8] Research from Finland, looking at the effect of dieting by comparing over 2,000 sets of twins, found that when one of the twins embarked on even a single attempt to lose weight, they then became between two and three times more likely to become overweight, when compared to their twin who did not attempt to diet.[9] The same effect is observed in children, between nine and fourteen years of age, where research into the eating patterns of over 17,000 children and adolescents found that dieting gave rise to a significantly increased risk of not only weight gain, but also binge eating.[10]

Dieting is counterproductive because it creates deprivation, making you want to eat more. It also takes no account of the reasons behind disordered eating in the first place. And until these have been addressed, any attempt to deal with the symptoms is doomed to failure.

What happens to children when they grow up in a house with dieting parents? Unsurprisingly, they model their behaviour (particularly girls and their mothers). Research tracking the eating habits of girls aged between seven and eleven and their mothers, over a two-year period, found that girls were significantly more likely to diet before the age of eleven if their mothers did so.[11] Given that dieting in childhood increases the risk of being overweight and of binge eating, it is not too great a leap to understand the effects of growing up in a 'dieting house'.

I grew up in such a house and my experiences echo the research precisely. My mother embarked on a 'healthy-living' regime when I was eight years old, joining a slimming club and starting regular aerobics classes. As a family, our eating changed almost overnight. Out went any 'bad' food, with biscuits, crisps, cakes, chocolate and the like all being banished from the house. Dessert was fruit or nothing, Sunday roasts were replaced with salads and eating out was curtailed. Ultimately, my mother was removing temptation from the house, and in its place came a huge set of scales for the bathroom and books and charts full of calorie-counting information. I was a healthy and happy eight-year-old – active, lean and a perfectly healthy weight for my age and height. But by the time I was nine years old I could tell you how many calories were in most foods and I had started my first diet. When I started puberty, my body began to change. I grew breasts and hips and began wearing a UK size twelve (US size eight). Looking back at photos of myself at that age I was clearly not fat, I just had curves. But I started to panic. I wasn't thin like some of my friends and the girls in the magazines I read. My mum encouraged me to join her on her diet when I was fourteen. I attended her old slimming club, lost two and a half stone and slimmed down to a UK size eight (US four). I can see now that this is when the problems that had begun when I was only nine years old really ramped up a gear. I began to eat in private, sneaking chocolate bars into my bedroom and hiding the wrappers, then I would feel guilty, so I wouldn't eat at all the next day. I spent my school lunch money on the forbidden 'treats' I was never allowed at home and would often eat two slices of cake for lunch, trying to 'save' calories for the 'naughty food' by not eating a sandwich or cooked meal. I yo-yoed between near starvation and bingeing for most of my teens. In my twenties, once I had left home, the disordered eating got worse. I would buy more and more of the food I hadn't been allowed at home, feeling guiltier with each mouthful, the shame causing me to binge more to try to palliate my feelings of self-doubt and disgust. This is a pattern that has continued throughout almost all my adult life, which saw me at seven stone overweight at my heaviest.

Twenty years on, I feel that I am just beginning to get a handle on my eating and finally feel in control. I have stopped dieting and jumping on all the new eating fads and 'lose-weight-quick' schemes. Instead, I have finally started listening to my body, responding to my feelings in a healthier way that doesn't involve food and, most importantly, I have stopped seeing food as something 'good' or 'bad'. Food is just food now; nothing is restricted, nothing is forbidden. For the first time since I was nine years old, I feel free. And I am determined to pass this freedom on to my own children. Now is the time to break the cycle of disordered eating that has passed down from generation to generation in my family. Do you feel ready to do the same?

Orthorexia

In 1996, American physician Steven Bratman coined the term 'orthorexia nervosa', or orthorexia for short. The term comes from the Greek words *'orthos'*, meaning correct or right, and *'orexi'* meaning appetite, and is roughly translated as 'correct appetite'. It is used to denote an unhealthy obsession with eating healthy food. The term is not used to apply to any ethical belief systems, religion or genuine food allergies or diseases leading to avoidance of specific foods, such as vegetarianism, veganism, kosher, halal or coeliac disease, but rather an obsession with restricting eating to only foods deemed entirely healthy. While, at first glance, orthorexia might seem healthy, the reality is quite the opposite. Bratman believes that this is an *unhealthy* eating pattern, causing individuals to suffer unintended negative consequences, such as social isolation, anxiety, a lack of instinctive eating and even malnutrition.

The Bratman orthorexia self-test

As no formal diagnostic criteria exist for orthorexia (it is not currently recognised in diagnostic manuals), Bratman has developed his own self-test – a simple list of six statements, as follows:[12]

1. I spend so much of my life thinking about, choosing and preparing healthy food that it interferes with other dimensions of my life, such as love, creativity, family, friendship, work and school.

2. When I eat any food I regard to be unhealthy, I feel anxious, guilty, impure, unclean and/or defiled; even to be near such foods disturbs me, and I feel judgemental of others who eat such foods.

3. My personal sense of peace, happiness, joy, safety and self-esteem is excessively dependent on the purity and rightness of what I eat.

4. Sometimes I would like to relax my self-imposed 'good-food' rules for a special occasion, such as a wedding or a meal with family or friends, but I find that I cannot. (Note: if you have a medical condition that makes it unsafe for you to make ANY exception to your diet, then this item does not apply.)

5. Over time, I have steadily eliminated more foods and expanded my list of food rules in an attempt to maintain or enhance health benefits; sometimes, I may take an existing food theory and add to it with beliefs of my own.

6. Following my theory of healthy eating has caused me to lose more weight than most people would say is good for me, or has caused other signs of malnutrition such as hair loss, loss of menstruation or skin problems.

Agreeing with *any* of these six statements, according to Bratman, could indicate the presence of orthorexia.

Orthorexia by proxy

Very little is known about orthorexia in children, as the idea is relatively new. The most important question to ask going forward, then, is how parental orthorexia impacts on the eating behaviour and beliefs of children – a concept often referred to as 'orthorexia by proxy'. Just as parental dieting can have a negative effect on the eating behaviour and weight of children, orthorexia is just as likely to impact negatively. If children grow up with a parent who is obsessed with all aspects of nutrition, completely restricting certain foods or even whole food groups, the chances are they will mimic this behaviour. As a consequence, they may grow up with anxiety around eating and experience difficulty integrating into certain social situations where food control is difficult, or sometimes impossible, or they may defy the parent's restrictions by bingeing and eating 'unhealthy' food in secret.

When parents have too much anxiety and obsess over what they feed their children, the children are bound to pick up on this. The difficulty is in striking a balance between modelling healthy eating habits and 'orthorexia by proxy'. So many parents judge their own worth, in part, by what their children do or don't eat. We are frequently attacked by the media for allowing our children to eat 'too much', be 'too picky' or not eat enough. Right from the beginning of our children's lives their weight is an issue. At baby clinics a parent will be praised if their baby has gained lots of weight, yet when the same child starts school, they will receive letters if he or she is even slightly above the recommended body mass index for their age.

While it is incredibly difficult to be the parent of a 'poor' eater, especially in a group full of 'good' eaters, it is hard to be the parent of the overweight child. Each week seems to bring about a change to governmental guidelines on how many vegetables we should eat and how much salt or sugar we should consume daily. One minute, we should eat margarine because butter is unhealthy, the next, butter is the order of the day. One day, fat is the enemy and 'low-fat' is all the rage, the next, sugar is the demon of the day. Is it any wonder that so many parents struggle with feeding their children, and that books such as this are necessary?

Parents would most likely do best by listening to their instincts and ignoring the conflicting advice, yet they are bombarded with new cookery books, celebrity nutrition experts, and an ever-increasing number of blogs and Instagram accounts about 'healthy eating'. The sad truth is, there is too much information available and this information overload erodes our confidence, creates a fear of food and makes our eating – and that of our children – disordered.

So how do we break this cycle? This is where gentle eating comes in. With this book, you can change your beliefs about eating and, in turn, make your child's eating something that is more mindful, more instinctive and altogether healthier. In Chapters 3 to 7, we will look at applying gentle-eating principles at different stages throughout childhood, from birth to teen. But before we do that, let's just take a look at reframing *your* attitude to food, with a quick reminder of some of the information we have covered in this chapter.

Tips on gentle eating for adults

- **Be mindful** Ask yourself why you are eating. Listen to your body's signals: if you are hungry, then eat; when you are full, stop eating.

- **Stop labelling food** Food is food. It doesn't have a personality. It isn't 'good' or 'naughty', 'healthy' or 'unhealthy'. A healthy diet is about all the components, not any one isolated food.

- **Detach emotions from eating** Recognise any tendencies you have to eat to try to regulate your emotions. Do you eat when you are stressed, angry, sad or bored? Once you recognise any patterns, you can work to find other ways to cope with these emotions that don't involve eating.

- **Reconsider social rules** There is no such thing as 'breakfast food' or 'dinner food'. And forget about prescribed mealtimes – if you're not hungry, don't eat just because it's lunchtime, and conversely, don't avoid eating if you are hungry, but it's not yet an appropriate time to eat. Also, don't eat because it is the socially acceptable thing to do. You can say 'no' to a slice of birthday cake in the office or the canapés at a party. It is not offensive to do so.

- **Don't diet** Don't restrict your portions if you are hungry and don't restrict certain food groups, especially if you really fancy something. No food should be forbidden. Try to resist jumping on the latest diet fad. They are all the same. They don't work, not long-term anyway, and they may even make you put on weight.

- **Don't use food as a reward** If you have had a good day, or achieved something and want to celebrate, you don't have to do it with food. Think of non-food ways to celebrate when something good happens.

- **Make friends with your body** You've been mean about your body for too long. Think about all the marvellous things it has accomplished. If you are a birth parent, think about the fact that you have created life with it. If you are an adoptive or foster parent, think about the nurturing and support you have given your child with it. Learn to appreciate, not criticise, your body and show it thanks and gratitude for the journey it has taken you on throughout your life so far.

- **Recognise patterns – and break them** Try to identify disordered eating behaviour acquired from your own childhood. Where do your beliefs come from? Try to understand why you behave in the way you do around food, recognising what and how you need to change.

- **Try to get enough sleep** Sleep is key in keeping your hormone levels stable, particularly ghrelin. Even the healthiest psychological approach to eating is going to be undermined by a persistent lack of sleep.

- **Avoid judging yourself by what your children eat** Your parenting should not be measured by how and what your children eat. Acknowledge what a brilliant parent you are and separate your relationship with your child from their eating.

We must work on ourselves first to break the disordered eating habits we have inherited and prevent them from carrying over into the next generation and the next. When we have understood our own relationship with food, we can move on to helping our children to develop gentle-eating habits. Ideally, you would begin right at the very start of life, from birth, which is why the next chapter is all about nutrition in the early weeks and months. If you have come to this book with an older child, however, you may wish to skip to the chapter relevant to their age.

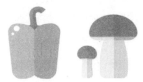

Chapter 3

Liquids Only – Birth to Six Months

While we, as parents, may be the biggest influence on our children's eating habits, the way they are first introduced to food is surely a close second. Many believe that our eating habits and relationships with food begin once we start to eat 'proper' food, or solids. However, the truth is, they begin far earlier than that: from the moment we are born and start to drink milk.

When a baby is born, the way they are fed can, and does, have a lasting impact on their eating habits and overall health for life. Gentle-eating principles – mindful, empowering, respectful and authoritative – apply from the very first day of your baby's life. Following them, even when your baby is on a milk-only diet, can help them to learn to self-regulate their eating from the outset and avoid many common eating issues later in life. If you are reading this book with a bump or a newborn, this chapter will help you to give your child the healthiest and, indeed, most gentle introduction to eating. If you have come to this book a little further down the line with your baby, know that it is never too late to start to feed in a more mindful, empowering, respectful and authoritative way, and that is exactly what this chapter will cover.

Your baby's microbiome and how it affects their eating

Before we look at gentle-eating principles and their implications in infancy, we must first consider an important concept that can and does affect your baby's eating behaviour, far beyond their birth: the microbiome.

Microbiome is the term used to describe the combined genetic code of the microbiota – or bacterial ecosystem – in the gut. The genes of the microbiome outnumber those in the rest of the body by around 100 to one and are of great importance to its functioning, playing a role in everything from nutrition to immunity. The microbiome also seems to play a significant role in obesity and feelings of satiation, with individuals with sub-optimal microbiomes being more likely to overeat and less likely to feel satiated. Therefore, in order to raise a child who is able to self-regulate their eating, we must consider any physiological elements that may get in the way of this.

Birth, breastfeeding and their impact on the microbiome

We acquire most of our microbiome at birth, when microbes begin to colonise our bodies. Prior to this – in utero – we are sterile, or free of microbes. The first microbes colonise a newborn baby courtesy of their mother: babies who are born vaginally are coated in a layer of microbes, transferred from the mother's vagina, these microbes help the baby to digest their first food – milk – as well as helping to provide them with some immunity to the new world they find themselves in. There is a significant difference between the microbiome of babies born vaginally, who are colonised by the 'good' bacteria found within their mother, and those born via Caesarean section, who miss out on a proportion of this colonisation, by bypassing the microbes in the mother's vagina and being born into a sterile surgical environment. Similarly, there is a difference between the microbiome of babies who have received antibiotics during the labour or birth and those who haven't.

Perhaps the best way to help to colonise your baby's microbiome with 'good' bacteria is to breastfeed. When mothers breastfeed, they share their own 'good' bacteria with their babies. Breast milk is a live substance that is constantly altering to provide optimal nutrition for the baby at any one point. While formula milk does contain bacteria, these can be harmful, which is why you should always make it up with boiling water, to kill any that may be in the milk powder.

Even if the baby is breastfed, however, the microbiome is still not optimal if the birth was via Caesarean. So is there anything else you can do to increase the health of your baby's microbiome? There are two options here – one that is pre-emptive in trying to prevent problems with the microbiome from the beginning (for anyone reading who is currently pregnant) and the other that can be used at any point in the child's life, no matter how long ago they were born. Let's look at both in a little more detail.

Protecting the microbiome in advance:
vaginal seeding

Vaginal seeding describes the process of transferring microbes found in the mother's vagina to the baby, by means of a rolled-up piece of sterile gauze which is inserted into the vagina for an hour before birth and then rubbed on the baby once they are born. The idea behind this is that the baby is still exposed to the beneficial bacteria found in the mother's vagina if they are born via Caesarean. The process is in the very early days of research, and understanding and evidence to date have proved rather contradictory. But many believe that it does show some promise.[1] Vaginal seeding does, however, carry risks. There is a chance that the mother may be carrying harmful bacteria and viruses, such as group B streptococcus and herpes simplex, that she is unaware of, and these may be passed on to the baby. This risk, however, is not unlike that posed to babies born vaginally.

Repairing the microbiome post birth:
probiotic supplements

Many believe that some of the 'good bacteria' missing at birth or eradicated due to antibiotics can in part be replaced using probiotics. These are supplements that contain amounts of certain live strains of the common gut bacterium, lactobacillus. Research has found a positive effect from the use of probiotics in babies in relation to a reduction in gastrointestinal problems[2] and eczema,[3] but as with vaginal seeding, significantly more evidence is needed as to their efficacy. Having said that, probiotic usage does not appear to present any risks and many parents decide that the chance of a positive effect on their child's microbiome is worth taking, as the supplements are relatively cheap to buy.

Making mindful choices about feeding methods

Mindful eating choices sit at the heart of gentle eating. When a baby is born, the choice of milk they are fed with is usually made by their parents. In order to uphold the gentle-eating tenets, parents need to be empowered to make their decision about feeding methods as informed as possible. This can be a tricky task, though, in societies flooded with aggressive marketing from formula manufacturers. Given the cost of a tin of formula-milk powder you would think that the cost of production is high. However, it is not the formula itself that costs a lot of money, but the marketing budgets of the manufacturers.[4] Simply put, the inflated price of infant formula milk funds the industry's business actions, which in turn keeps the price high.

In contrast, funding for breastfeeding support and education is woefully low. To increase breastfeeding rates, a far greater budget needs to be devoted to educating all health professionals who come into contact with new families. Currently, understanding of breastfeeding among family doctors is low; most receive less than one day's education on breastfeeding in their medical training, even though research has shown that specific training makes a big difference to the understanding and advice given.[5] Too often, medical professionals give conflicting breastfeeding advice, or guidance based upon their own personal experiences and opinions, or, more worrying still, information received from formula manufacturers.

I was once asked to speak at a conference for a well-known and respected nursing and midwifery journal and excitedly accepted the invitation. Upon arrival at the conference, I walked through an exhibition area and immediately found myself facing not one, but three formula-milk manufacturers, each of them offering free gifts to the midwives and health visitors in attendance, given out by pushy sales representatives eager to talk about the benefits of their products and why the health professionals should recommend them to parents. New parents, believing that the information given to them by medical professionals should be entirely trustworthy, are understandably confused. Often, poor advice results in the eventual failure of breastfeeding when there was no underlying physiological or any other reason why it could not have continued. Perhaps the saddest aspect of this failure on the part of health professionals to give evidence-based advice, coupled with inadequate support, is that parents who make the decision to switch to formula milk are racked with guilt and disappointment and the feeling that it is they themselves who have somehow 'failed'. They don't see that they have *been* failed. It is simply not their fault. This categorically should not happen. Parents should receive appropriate support to feed their baby as they prefer. In a utopian society, formula manufacturers would be banned from using heavy-handed and unethical marketing strategies, and health professionals would be well trained and non-biased. Sadly, we are not there yet.

How to find good, reliable information and advice about infant feeding

While seeking opinions and guidance about breastfeeding from medical staff may seem the best approach, in reality it is not. There are many passionate, dedicated and well-informed midwives and health visitors who give excellent breastfeeding advice, but there are also many who do not. The hard task for a new parent is to try to deduce into which category their medical caregiver fits. There is no easy answer here. Instinct is perhaps the best clue. If you feel uncomfortable with the advice, or if it is unsuccessful, perhaps the most empowering and mindful step you can take is to approach a lactation consultant or breastfeeding counsellor. Both are trained professionals who have studied the intricacies of breastfeeding for years and are aware of the latest research. It is usually possible to access a breastfeeding counsellor for free, either face to face, or via a telephone or Internet consultation. Lactation consultants, on the other hand, generally charge for their services, although their fee is usually more than worth it. Lactation consultants and breastfeeding counsellors can provide advice on bottle-feeding too, and can be very helpful if you are struggling with bottle-feeding your baby. (See page 205 for a list of infant-feeding resources, including information on where to find a breastfeeding counsellor or lactation consultant.)

Gentle-eating alternatives to breastfeeding

There is an assumption in society that the only two choices when it comes to feeding babies are to breastfeed or to bottle-feed with formula milk. There are, however, several other options, as recommended by the World Health Organization,[6] before giving formula milk in a bottle. The preference for feeding methods is as follows (from most to least preferable):

- Breastfeeding directly from the baby's own mother

- Milk from the baby's own mother, expressed rather than direct from the breast, then given from a cup, bottle, syringe or supplementary nursing system (see below)

- Milk from a wet nurse – breastfeeding from a lactating woman who is not the mother

- Milk from a milk bank – breast milk from another woman, expressed

- Breast-milk substitute, formula milk – fed by cup, rather than a bottle

- Breast-milk substitute – formula milk, fed by bottle

Up until a century ago, wet nursing was the main – indeed, only – healthy alternative to breastfeeding. Feeding directly from the breast allows the baby to control the flow of milk much more than if the donor milk was expressed and given by bottle, which is why wet nursing is considered preferable to using donor milk. When a baby is able to control the flow of milk themselves they can regulate their food intake and satiety levels. As we know, this empowerment and self-regulation are an important part of gentle eating. It is possible, however, to simulate breast-feeding while using donor milk via the use of a supplementary nursing system (SNS) – an invention which allows a mother to feed her baby milk at the breast, and which can be particularly helpful if there are milk supply issues or the baby has difficulty sucking. An SNS includes a pouch which holds milk and fine tubing which carries the milk to the mother's nipple, allowing the baby to take both the nipple and tubing into the mouth to feed, encouraging a sucking motion and getting them to work for the feed, as they would with a normal breastfeed. If an SNS is not used, then the next option is to feed the baby expressed or human donor milk via a special small, open-top cup instead of a bottle. Cup-feeding allows the baby to pace their own feeding and to 'lap' up the milk with their tongue, a little like a kitten or a puppy may do. This means that the baby is more actively involved in the feeding process than they are with a bottle and, importantly, allows them more control over the feeding. Once again, this control encourages the baby to self-regulate their food intake from very early on, which can have a very positive impact on their regulation of eating as they grow. If donor milk is not available, then SNS and cup-feeding also work with formula milk. The pacing and control they offer may help to cancel out some of the negative effects of using formula milk, by avoiding bottles and empowering the baby to take more control over their eating experience. In fact, it could be argued that this is far more important than the type of milk consumed.

Choosing formula milk

If you visit Internet discussion groups, there is often a lot of chatter about what formula milk is 'best for babies'. Many parents will buy a brand because it has the word 'organic' in the title, because it is the most expensive brand or because the advertising states it is 'closest to breast milk'. The good news for parents who formula-feed their babies is that there are very strict regulations about the content of infant milk. In the UK, they are known as 'the Infant Formula and Follow-on Formula regulations'[7] and they specify the core ingredients and amounts contained in different stages of milk. Thus, there is very little difference between the various milks available and those differences are really just down to marketing. Similarly, 'closest to breast milk' is a red herring. Although the important key ingredients remain the same, breast milk is ever changing, is different for each baby and changes regularly as the baby grows. Breast milk contains over 300 different ingredients compared to the seventy-five in formula milk. With all this in mind, the most sensible choice is to simply buy the cheapest formula milk. Ironically, charging a higher price is often part of the marketing strategy of certain companies, as it fools parents into thinking the product must be better than that of cheaper competitors if it is more expensive. But more expensive doesn't mean better; it just means that you're contributing towards the manufacturer's marketing budget. So, you can save your money, safe in the knowledge that the regulations are there to protect you, and the different brands really are all the same.

When to move up to a different stage of formula milk

After the confusion of different brands all claiming different health benefits comes the uncertainty around 'moving up' a stage – that is, changing to milk products aimed at different ages.

Stage one is the starting point. Stage-one formula is a 'first milk' that can be used from birth. Made from cow's milk, it consists of two different proteins, casein and whey. However, there is significantly more whey than casein, as whey is believed to be easier to digest. Hungry-baby milk, also used from birth, simply has a higher casein content, making it harder to digest, the assumption being that it keeps babies 'fuller for longer' (a claim that is not backed by any evidence).

Stage-two formula, or 'follow-on milk', is used from six months of age. There is no benefit to switching to follow-on milk for the baby; it is purely a marketing ploy to circumvent the ban on advertising formula milk for under-six-month-olds. (Often companies will use babies who look younger than six months in their adverts, to suggest to viewers and readers that their brand of milk is a good choice for younger babies too.) Stage-three milk, used from twelve months, is again unnecessary. It is another marketing ploy to keep parents buying formula milk for longer than necessary. Babies older than twelve months no longer need formula milk; however, this would mean a huge loss of income for the formula manufacturers, so they market a milk specifically for toddlers, implying that it is better for them than cow's milk. It isn't. There is no reason to change a baby from their original first-stage milk. In fact, it is likely *better* for them to stay on it until they reach twelve months of age and then switch to much cheaper full-fat cow's milk.

How to bottle-feed in the best way possible

While breastfeeding naturally follows gentle-eating principles – that is, the baby is always in control of the pace of feeding and when it ends – if you are using a bottle to feed your baby, there are a few simple steps that you can take to make the feeding process the best it can be for your child. These incorporate gentle-eating principles and help to make the act as nurturing and enjoyable as possible for both parent and child.

1. Ignore the clock

Often formula-feeding is linked heavily with feeding to a schedule, an idea that is not in line with mindful and respectful eating. This really doesn't have to be the case though. It is completely possible to bottle-feed on demand, following the same principle as breastfeeding. Demand feeding is all about being aware of your baby's hunger cues, particularly the early ones (a point we will discuss later in this chapter – see page 60). It is a little harder to respond as quickly when you are bottle-feeding as you must make the formula and cool or warm it to the correct temperature, which takes time. However, with a little bit of advanced planning and learning your baby's early hunger cues, it should be possible to respond fairly quickly.

A clock, formula tin or book cannot ever tell you when a baby will be hungry, in much the same way that socially dictated mealtimes often don't correlate with our own hunger. Only the baby knows when they are hungry. Sometimes they will need feeding again soon after a feed; at other times they will go for much longer periods without wanting another feed. The key here is to be flexible and responsive, respecting their natural appetite.

2. Watch the baby not the bottle

Just as hunger cannot be measured by a chart or printed instructions, neither can satiety. Only the baby knows when they have had enough milk. The formula packaging may be able to give you a rough guide to the amount of milk your baby may drink at a given age, but it is only that – a guide. Your baby may be particularly hungry at one feed and less so at another. Don't expect them to always take the same amount at each feed. We don't eat the same amount at every meal, so why would a baby be any different? Being mindful when bottle-feeding means being aware of your baby's satiety signals and carefully watching for when they have had enough milk. Don't be tempted to try to get them to take more to finish the bottle. This is a little like our adult obsession with 'clearing your plate', and it doesn't encourage healthy eating habits.

3. Get some skin-to-skin

Breastfeeding provides Mum and baby with skin-to-skin contact, which is known to stimulate the secretion of the bonding and calming hormone oxytocin. Bottle-feeding often means holding a fully clothed baby on a fully clothed chest, which means no skin-to-skin contact. There is, however, no reason why you cannot enjoy the same contact when bottle-feeding. Undo some buttons on your shirt or lift your shirt up and hold your baby on your bare skin, close to your chest. And this isn't just for mums. Partners can do this too, meaning all caregivers can enjoy the chemical benefits of skin-to-skin contact that is so often needlessly reserved for breastfeeding mothers.

4. Let the baby take the bottle

When breastfeeding, it is the baby who decides to latch onto the breast to begin feeding, whereas bottle-feeding is usually begun by a parent inserting a bottle into the baby's mouth. To make feeding more baby-led and respectful, begin feeding by holding the bottle teat close to your baby's cheek and waiting for them to turn and latch onto it, pulling it into their mouths themselves. Similarly, when you feel your baby trying to push the teat out of their mouth, take it out immediately and wait for them to latch on again to restart.

5. Be mindful

Eating mindfully is one of the key principles of gentle eating, but being mindful of the moment while feeding your baby is important too. Far too often parents bottle-feed on the go, or multitask, feeding while concentrating on something else. When you do this, you can never be truly respectful of your baby's eating. So, when your baby feeds, as often as possible, really take time to just 'be'. Be still, hug them, talk to them, stroke their legs and their arms, smell their head, feel the weight of them in your arms and just take time out from your everyday life to enjoy the moment. Soon your baby will be on the move and these sweet milk feeds will be a thing of the past. Don't be tempted to multitask and check texts or emails or make a phone call when you are feeding your baby, and especially never prop a bottle. Treat it as a time that is as much about bonding and connection as it is about nourishment.

6. Hold your baby in a more upright position

Many people tend to bottle-feed their babies in a horizontal position, with the baby lying down in their lap or in their arms. When babies are breastfed, in contrast, they are held in a more upright, almost seated position, which some believe can reduce the incidence of ear infections and aid digestion. A good rule of thumb is to hold your baby just upright enough that the bottle is being held horizontal with the floor.

7. Respect your baby's pauses

When babies breastfeed, they tend to feed for a while and then stop, take a rest, look around and so on, then they feed again and pause again. Helping your baby to do the same with a bottle can help to slow feeding down and enable them to recognise their satiety signals, reducing overeating. After you have satiated their immediate hunger with the bottle, encourage them to stop and 'chat' with you, smile at each other, have a cuddle and so on. Gently winding them by rubbing their back or shifting position every five or ten minutes or so can encourage this, as can changing the side on which you are supporting them, i.e. switching from your left arm to your right.

8. Use a slow-flow teat

Bottle teats usually encourage a much faster flow of milk than breastfeeding, which can cause the baby to take in more milk than they need, especially as they don't have to work very hard to get it, unlike breastfed babies. Switching to a slow-flow teat allows the baby to control the flow of milk more and naturally slows the feeding, thus preventing overeating.

The problem with feeding schedules

As soon as you have a baby, you quickly become bombarded with advice, often unsolicited, to 'get the baby on a schedule'. Many childcare experts and workers recommend that babies should feed at strict times and sleep at others. These routines are said to reduce crankiness, bad habits and sleep problems. In reality, none of this is true. By dictating when and how much a baby should eat we totally override their innate hunger and satiety cues. Scheduling feeds disrespects their needs in an attempt to meet our own. While research has shown that feeding to a schedule results in higher maternal wellbeing, it has a bad effect on the child's development, causing poorer cognitive functioning and even impacting negatively on academic achievement later in life.[8] In addition, restricting feeds (by timing them and controlling amounts) has been shown to be associated with a higher body weight in later life.[9]

In contrast, feeding a baby 'on demand' (a rather negative-sounding term that really just means that the parents are mindful of the baby's levels of hunger and satiety and offer food when the baby is hungry, not by the clock) is significantly better for children. Feeding on demand ensures that the baby is in control of their feeding right from the very start of life.

Not only do they quickly recognise when they are hungry and have their needs met by their carers, they learn, importantly, when they are full and are not forced to eat when they are not hungry. For this reason, the World Health Organization recommends that babies are fed 'on demand'.[10] This method of feeding encourages parents to be mindful of their baby's hunger and satiety signals, which allows them to fulfil the other three principles of gentle eating – respecting their baby's hunger and satiety, empowering the baby to follow their own cues and feeding in an authoritative way that gives as much control to the baby as possible.

Responsive feeding

Feeding on demand in infancy provides the groundwork for something known as 'responsive feeding'. This is a way of feeding children, no matter their age, that puts them in the driving seat and in control of their own bodily needs. Responsive feeding enables children to recognise and respond to their own feelings of hunger and satiety and helps them to be mindful of their body's needs concerning food. Responsive feeding is the key to facilitating self-regulation surrounding food from the very beginning of life. Research has shown that responsive feeding beginning in infancy is associated with the healthiest patterns in eating as children grow.[11] In essence, it is what gentle eating is all about: being mindful, empowering, respectful and authoritative. Whether you are feeding a newborn, a six-month-old, a toddler, an eight-year-old or a teenager, the idea of being responsive to their needs is always key to raising children who have a healthy relationship with food.

Hunger and satiety cues

In Chapter 1, we looked at the hunger and satiety cycle and how gentle eating relies on the individual recognising and responding to their bodily signals. Observational studies have shown that despite their lack of speech, babies have a sophisticated range of ways – an astounding total of twenty-two – in which they communicate their hunger and satiety,[12] and if parents are to practise gentle eating with their babies, they must learn to understand these. The following table highlights the most common hunger and satiety signals:

Signs of hunger	Signs of satiety
Turning head to one side	'Soft hands' (hands relax, slightly open)
Opening and closing mouth ('rooting')	Body relaxing (feels softer and heavier)
Squirming/wriggling/stretching	Face (especially forehead and cheeks) relaxing
Sticking tongue out/smacking lips	Arms dropping to side of body
Bringing hands to mouth	Sucking slowing, pausing more often
Crying (the very latest sign of hunger)	Falling asleep

These cues can be observed from the very first day of your baby's life, and learning to 'read' and act on them as much as possible will help you to begin to take a responsive role, following the ethos of gentle eating, from the start.

Feeding in the night

There is a tremendous amount of confusing advice available concerning night-time parenting of babies. Parents can understandably feel overwhelmed and anxious concerning their child's sleep and when it becomes problematic to continue to feed at night. In the UK, the National Health Service (NHS) website states that night feeds are usually no longer needed after six months of age.[13] However, this is not an evidence-based claim. While most babies are developed enough, with a sufficiently large stomach capacity to last for eight to twelve hours overnight without a feed, this completely ignores any individuality with regards to hunger. Some babies will need milk in the night because they have consumed less in the day, something that is especially common for breastfed babies who have been separated from their mother in the daytime. In this instance, they will often need to feed several times in the night – something known as 'reverse cycling'. Others may not have eaten much in the day or at bedtime because they have been ill, or are experiencing teething pain. Some may not have consumed much milk in the daytime because they have been eating solid foods and others may be thirsty, rather than hungry. We tend to overlook thirst as a legitimate need at night. Experts commonly believe that night feeds are unnecessary after six months as the baby 'can't possibly be that hungry', but it is important to understand that milk to a baby, especially breast milk, quenches thirst as well as resolving hunger. Thirst is often increased in the night if it is hot. Summer, in particular, often sees more night feeding than in the colder months. Thirst is also increased if the humidity in the room is low, perhaps from air conditioning or central heating, something which is exacerbated if the baby is a mouth breather. Many adults take a glass of water to bed with them, so that when they wake in the night with a dry throat they can take a sip or two. Babies need this too. You are not encouraging 'bad habits' when you respond to your baby's need for nutrition in the night, as many mistakenly believe. The responsive way to view night feeds is that if the baby believes that they need to drink, we should trust them.

Centile concerns

Trusting your baby to regulate their own feeding is fairly easy when they are moving up the weight and height centiles or tracking along on the fiftieth. But when they deviate from the charts, particularly falling from them, or they track along on the second centile, it can be very different. Research has found that over 70 per cent of parents misinterpret centile charts and are easily confused by their findings.[14] Centile charts can make it easy to second-guess your parenting, making you wonder if you really are doing what's best for your child. And remarks from well-meaning but interfering people about your child's frame, suggesting that they need to be fed more or started on solids to 'build them up', can also cause a great deal of anxiety, especially if you have friends or family with similar-aged babies who are adhering to a high centile or climbing through them.

The reality is, however, that it is OK for your baby to be above or lower than the average – somebody must be! It's OK for them to be on the second centile and it's OK for them to be on the ninety-eighth. As adults, we're not all exactly the same height and weight; similarly, not sticking exactly to the centile line is not a disaster. Growth isn't precisely linear. Sometimes babies will have spurts of growing quickly; sometimes they will slow down for a bit. Babies who are mobile and active may well show slower gains in comparison to babies of a similar age who are immobile. Bouts of minor illness can also have a temporary effect on the growth trajectory. So while centile charts may be a useful tool, they are not the sole predictor (or an infallible one) for gauging health. They are not an indicator that parents need to take over control of the baby's eating by restricting or increasing feeds irrespective of the baby's appetite. Similarly, they don't indicate that a baby needs to be weaned onto solids early. More than anything, however, they are not a reflection of 'good' or 'bad' parenting. Centile information provides just one piece of the puzzle regarding a child's health status and should not be taken in isolation, either by parents or health professionals.

Feeding away from Mum

Sometimes a baby's separation from their mother is unavoidable and sometimes it is encouraged, even if the mother is available. Some of the most frequently asked questions surrounding the early weeks and months concern feeding a baby in the absence of their mother and how fathers can best bond with their baby at these times. Let's look at how parents can respond in a gentle, mindful and respectful way in such circumstances.

How do you get a breastfed baby to take a bottle?

There seems to be a pervasive myth that a breastfed baby should get used to taking a bottle as soon as possible, the idea being that it will encourage them to learn to fall asleep without the breast. This is not true. Gentle eating is about working at the baby's own pace and following their cues, to enable them to take control of their own eating. There is no rush to create sleep independent of breastfeeding, or to introduce a bottle, unless it is something that you really need to do. If, however, you need to be separated from your baby at some point in the not too distant future, what do you do if they are not keen on taking a bottle? The following tips may help:

- Start your attempts a good couple of weeks before you need to. Don't leave it until the day that you have to be away.

- Look for a bottle teat that is wide at the base, reminiscent of the breast areola. When babies latch onto the breast their lips splay much wider than do those of babies who bottle-feed and tend to purse their lips due to the much narrower bottle teat.

- Go for a slow-flow teat, as this is the most like breastfeeding. Breastfed babies need to work to get milk and when they do, they control it. This means many bottle teats are too fast-flowing for them.

- Let somebody else offer the bottle. When you are practising in advance of leaving your baby, bottle-feeding is often more successful if somebody other than the mother does it. Sometimes babies can get distracted if the mother is even in the same room.

- Offer the bottle at the very earliest sign of hunger, when the baby is still calm. Don't wait until they are upset and start to cry – this is a late hunger cue and they are likely to get more worked up when they are offered a bottle at this stage.

- The coldness of a bottle teat can be an uncomfortable change for babies and may put them off. Try gently warming the bottle teat in warm water for a minute before feeding, to mimic the warmth of the breast. When babies breastfeed, the areola and nipple are obviously warm – 37°C, to be precise.

- Follow the baby-led bottle-feeding guidelines on page 54 and try different positions. Some babies prefer to be seated completely upright, others slightly reclined.

- If you are not having any success with the bottle, it may be better to switch to a cup or spoon or even a syringe to feed the baby. If you're using a cup or spoon, hold them close to the baby's mouth and allow them to lap up the milk. If you are using a syringe, squirt very small amounts of milk into the mouth at a time, allowing plenty of pauses for the baby to swallow and rest.

- If you are using expressed breast milk and none of the previous tips work, then there may be an issue with the milk itself. Some women produce an excess of lipase – an enzyme that assists in the breakdown of fat in the milk to aid digestion. An excess of lipase can cause milk to taste soapy when the milk is refrigerated or frozen and may cause babies to reject expressed milk. A simple way to check if this may be the case is to taste the milk yourself; if excess lipase is an issue it should be easy to detect. It is possible to heat the milk to just shy of boiling point, or scorching, which will inactivate the lipase and hopefully improve the taste. If this is still unsuccessful, then donor or formula milk may be the best alternative.

Sometimes, despite the best planning, babies end up taking very little milk when away from their mothers. The general consensus here – and my personal experience certainly bears this out – is that they will eat if they are really hungry. However, what usually happens is that the baby makes up for the lack of feeding as soon as the mother returns. For instance, if the mother is away all day, then the baby will likely feed very regularly in the evening and throughout the night, so-called 'reverse cycling'. This is a completely normal and healthy feeding pattern, and certainly not a 'sleep problem' as some may believe. Reverse cycling is not solely about nutrition, however; it also provides an important opportunity for mother and baby to rebond after a period of separation.

Can dads bond with their baby without giving them a bottle?

At birth, the bond between baby and mother is already nine months old. The baby learns to recognise his mother's voice and the sound of her heartbeat while still in utero, while the mother learns to understand his likes and dislikes, sleep and wake patterns. As soon as he is born he begins to differentiate the smell of his mother over and above any other scent. The touch of his mother's skin on his triggers the release of a cascade of hormone that calm him and help to regulate his temperature and breathing. If the mother is breastfeeding, the baby associates her with meeting all his needs. The baby is often only calmed when he is at the breast therefore dads can feel helpless, unable to soothe their own child or relieve some of the pressure on their partner for a while. Consequently, a breastfeeding mother and baby can sometimes seem like an impenetrable unit and dads, understandably, can feel a little on the back foot when it comes to bonding.

The most common advice is for the dad to 'give the baby a bottle or two' – the assumption here being that for bonding to take place, feeding is required. The truth is that it really isn't. The work of American psychologist Harry Harlow, and his experiments with attachment in monkeys in the 1950s, disproved the previously held theory of 'cupboard love'.[15] Cupboard love was believed to occur when a child formed a conditional bond with the individual who fed them. Therefore, if a mother was breastfeeding, it was believed that the baby would love her more than his father because of the provision of food. Even though this theory was shattered long ago, it still prevails almost as strongly in society today as it did in the 1950s. While dads may feel good about being able to nourish their baby physically, there are many ways they can nourish them emotionally, which is perhaps more important (see box opposite).

OTHER WAYS DADS CAN BOND WITH BABY

There are so many wonderful ways for a dad to bond with his baby that don't involve feeding. Here are a few examples:

- **Babywearing** Nothing is more amazing for a father than to hold their baby close to their chest, in a supportive baby sling or carrier. This close, prolonged contact enables fathers to nuzzle their baby's head and talk softly to them, leaving their arms free to get on with other things. My own husband particularly loved the attention he got while carrying our babies in public, showing off both the babies and the sling!
- **Skin-to-skin contact** Naked, or at least topless, cuddles are amazing. They generate the release of oxytocin (the love hormone) in both father and child, who get to know each other through touch and smell, as well as sight. This can also be a wonderful way of soothing a fractious baby.
- **Co-bathing** Sharing a bath with a baby is such a special experience. It enables skin-to-skin contact, while holding your baby in warm water – a state reminiscent for babies of being in the uterus, and one which is calming for them. Observing just how much your baby enjoys the experience is one of the best parts of being a new parent.
- **Baby massage** This is wonderful for relaxing babies and parents alike. Again, it stimulates the release of oxytocin and reduces stress hormones. It's a great way for fathers to get to know their baby by touch and helps with their sleep too. →

- **Reading** Reading books to babies is an amazing thing to do. It helps to build a real connection and a love of books for life, as well as forming a vital part of a good bedtime ritual. Combining bedtime stories, massage and co-bathing creates an optimal bedtime routine which can be a special task for fathers each evening, before the final input from Mum when she feeds the baby to sleep.
- **Practical care** Changing nappies, winding and dressing may seem like boring, mundane tasks, but they all provide wonderful opportunities to bond with babies. Talking or singing as they dress or wipe little bottoms brings fathers closer to their babies and helps to build a lasting relationship of trust.

Any one of the above activities can provide bonding that is equal to giving a bottle of milk; combining two or three of them provides a far superior bonding experience.

Before we end this chapter, let's remind ourselves of how the gentle-eating principles apply right from the very start of life. Gentle-eating principles in infancy mean parents making mindful and informed decisions about the milk that they feed their baby and how they feed it. Respect is shown to the baby by observing, identifying and following their hunger and satiety cues, and the baby is empowered to take as much control of the feeding process as possible, whether through breastfeeding 'on demand', using a cup or SNS or by following baby-led bottle-feeding principles. By adopting an authoritative stance to milk feeds, allowing the baby to lead, parents naturally embrace gentle eating.

The early months of life provide the groundwork for gentle eating in the months and years to follow. That doesn't mean, however, that if you started feeding your child in a different way, it is too late to implement gentle-eating principles and reap the rewards. In each of the following chapters we will consider eating at different ages, including how to change to a gentle-eating approach if you began feeding your child in a more authoritarian way. Let's move on now to older babies and, specifically, their first experiences of solid food.

Chapter 4

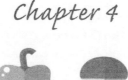

Introducing Solids – Six to Twelve Months

I ntroducing solids, or 'weaning', as it is more commonly known, is an exciting time for parents and babies alike. If gentle-eating principles are applied from the very start, they allow you to enjoy the process, knowing that you are giving your baby the most empowering and respectful start to their journey towards eating solid food. If you have come to this chapter having already started to wean your baby, then be assured that it is never too late to switch to a gentler style of weaning.

Let's remind ourselves of the gentle-eating principles once again, before discussing how they apply to introducing solids. Gentle eating is:

- mindful

- empowering

- respectful

- authoritative.

What does this look like when applied to babies of weaning age?

First, it means that as parents and carers, we are mindful of the abilities of our children both psychologically and physiologically, and of how the whole eating process affects them. In addition, we are mindful of the science and evidence surrounding eating in babies and the introduction of solids. The decisions we make concerning weaning are informed ones.

Next, we view weaning as being empowering for babies. We are led by them, from the timing of when it starts, to how much they eat, what they eat and how they eat. Weaning following gentle-eating principles is about putting babies in control as much as possible and starting on the path to empowering them to trust their own satiety and hunger cues.

Respect is central to weaning. The respect parents have for their babies helps them to sit back and trust them, knowing that respect at an early age is one of the best ways to create healthy eating habits for life.

This is all summarised as an authoritative parenting style. Authoritative parents are nurturing and empathic. They are informed and eager to let their children take control over aspects of their lives that are age appropriate. They naturally support a responsive-feeding style and encourage children to follow their own hunger and satiety cues by showing that they trust them.

But how does all this look in reality? It starts with placing the decision to start weaning in the baby's hands as much as possible and follows from there.

When should you wean onto solids?

Weaning has had a fairly erratic history throughout the years. At the start of the twentieth century, parents were advised to keep their babies on a liquid-only diet until they were twelve months of age. They were advised to supplement breast milk with cod-liver oil to prevent rickets and orange juice to prevent scurvy.[1] In the 1930s, the weaning age was brought forward because of concerns that babies were not getting enough nutrients. The age became ever younger after this, and by the 1970s most babies were fully weaned onto solid foods by four months of age, with many starting much earlier. It was not uncommon to feed a month-old baby a bottle of milk containing cereals, or to give a two-month-old baby a rusk to suck on. In 1994, the UK's Department of Health declared that the ideal window to begin weaning onto solids was between four and six months of age.[2] This advice was commonly misinterpreted, however, and many healthcare professionals recommended that weaning should begin when the baby was four months, or sixteen weeks, old. Indeed, when my first child was born in 2002, I was told by my health visitor that he should be weaned as soon as he was sixteen weeks old because he weighed 10lb at birth and 'wouldn't be able to wait any longer'. I know now that this was incorrect and that she had misinterpreted the guidelines. However, as a first-time mother, I had no reason to question the words of an experienced health professional.

My own experience of weaning advice given at the start of the twenty-first century was backed up by research conducted in 2000 showing that most babies were weaned onto solids by seventeen weeks of age.[3] But by 2005, the average age of weaning onto solids had increased to nineteen weeks, or just before five months. This figure is more in line with the World Health Organization's recommendation of around six months, or rather that babies should be exclusively breastfed for the first six months[4] – advice that was echoed by the UK Department of Health in 2003, which stated that 'Breastfeeding is the best form of nutrition for infants. Exclusive breastfeeding is recommended for the first six months (26 weeks) of an infant's life as it provides all the nutrients a baby needs.' In 2008, the European Food Safety Authority (EFSA) stated that exclusive breastfeeding for six months was a desirable goal and that weaning onto solids should begin by six months, but not before four.[5] 'Around six months' seems to be the most sensible guideline, although this does not mean that parents must wait until the day their baby turns six months old to begin weaning, nor does it mean that all babies will be ready to wean at that age. In all cases, the ultimate guide should always be the needs and readiness of the individual baby.

When is milk alone not enough?

Undoubtedly, the guiding force behind the change in opinion as to the 'proper' age for weaning in recent years has been a greater scientific understanding of the nutritional needs of babies. We are now able to research the impact, both short and long term, of the age of weaning and – importantly – when they need something other than milk to stay healthy.

The major assumption underlying the advice that babies should be weaned onto solid food at around six months is that milk alone is not enough nutritionally beyond this age. The World Health Organization (WHO) state that the age of weaning is the time when most babies are at risk of malnutrition, although not necessarily because milk cannot provide all the baby's needs, but rather because weaning means a reduction in milk intake.

The following table provides an insight into the nutrients provided by breast milk and the percentage of the recommended daily allowance for babies aged six and twelve months of age.[6]

Nutrient	Average per 100ml of breast milk	Percentage of RDA of all milk feeds at six months (875ml)	Percentage of RDA of all milk feeds at twelve months (550ml)
Energy KJ	280	99%	48%
Energy Kcal	67	99%	48%
Protein (g)	1.3	100%	65%
Fat (g)	4.2	100%	100%
Carbohydrate (g)	7	100%	100%
Calcium (mg)	35	100%	39%
Iron (mcg)	76	6%	4%
Vitamin A (mcg)	60	100%	66%
Vitamin C (mg)	3.8	83%	35%
Vitamin D (mcg)	0.01	10%	10%

This table helps us to see that most of a baby's nutrient needs are met solely by breast milk, until they are six months of age. After this, although breast milk does not deliver all their nutritional requirements, it still provides a significant proportion and that remains the case until their first birthday. There are, however, two nutrients that are not supplied in sufficient quantities by breast milk alone: iron and vitamin D. You may have been shocked by the low percentages for both of these, but we will look at them in a little more detail and you will find that the figures are not as alarming as they might seem.

Iron needs in infancy

Babies are born with stores of enough iron to last approximately six months.[7] Therefore, iron deficiency before this point is highly unlikely in an otherwise healthy baby. Research has shown that the risk of iron-deficiency anaemia is significantly lower for babies who experienced delayed cord clamping post birth, compared to those who didn't.[8] Delayed cord clamping lets the umbilical cord finish pulsating before it is cut, allowing the baby's full blood volume to return to their body from the placenta and umbilical cord. If the umbilical cord is cut while it is pulsating, the baby's blood volume will be incomplete, with some still circulating in the placenta and cord.

In addition to the baby's natural stores, they also receive some iron from milk. While breast milk may contain very little iron, what it does contain is readily absorbed by the body, at a 50–70 per cent rate. In comparison, iron-fortified formula milk may appear to provide a baby with significantly more iron, however its absorption by the body is poor, at a rate of only 3–12 per cent. Iron in regular cow's milk has an absorption rate of around 10 per cent, considerably lower than that from human milk.[9] As the baby moves into their second six months of life and their iron stores begin to decrease, they will need it from a source other than milk, although the high absorption rate from breast milk somewhat negates the low content for breastfed babies. Iron in solid food takes one of two forms: heme iron, found in meats, and non-heme iron, found in plants. Heme iron is more easily absorbed by the body, at a rate of around 15 per cent, compared with 7–11 per cent for non-heme.[10]

Vitamin D in infancy

Vitamin D is an essential vitamin that controls the uptake of calcium in our blood. It is therefore essential for the growth of healthy bones, with a deficiency causing the disease rickets. Most of our vitamin D doesn't come from our food but from exposure to sunlight, which causes our skin to create it. In fact, we consume very little vitamin D through our diets, the little we get coming mainly from eggs and oily fish. While infant formula milks are fortified with vitamin D, breast milk is naturally low in it. In order to get enough vitamin D from sunlight exposure, we need to be exposed to sun that is high in the sky – something that usually only occurs in the summer months in most countries. Many public-health authorities therefore recommend that vitamin D is supplemented. Public Health England recommend that adults and children over the age of one year should consider taking a daily supplement containing 10mcg of vitamin D, particularly during autumn and winter.[11] The UK's Department of Health recommends that all children aged six months to five years are given vitamin supplements containing vitamins A, C and D every day and that babies who are being breastfed are given a daily vitamin D supplement from birth.[12] This recommendation is echoed by the American Academy of Pediatrics, which suggests that all babies should receive 400IU of vitamin D per day and that all breastfed babies should be supplemented from birth.[13]

When is the digestive system ready for solids?

During the first three or four months of life, a baby's easy-to-digest milk diet doesn't require salivary amylase (the enzyme that enables the body to convert starch to sugar in order to then convert food to energy). Production of the enzyme begins and slowly increases over their first six months, reaching levels comparable with an adult's by around five to six months of age. It is only at this point that babies can convert the nutrients found in starchy foods (such as cereals, fruit and vegetables) into energy. If babies are weaned onto solids before this age, their nutrient absorption will be significantly poorer and can lead to them developing digestive disturbances such as diarrhoea, constipation and stomach cramps. In addition, early weaning has been linked to a higher risk of obesity, coeliac disease, diabetes and eczema,[14] with research showing no benefit in introducing additional foods before four to six months.[15]

Weaning onto solids for babies at risk of allergies

The NHS advises that potential allergenic foods (such as eggs, shellfish, nuts and wheat) should be introduced one at a time, from six months. Introducing them in this way allows parents to deduce what has caused any reaction more easily.[16] Allergy UK advises that babies at risk of certain allergies, such as those with a family history, should ideally be breastfed and weaned onto solids at around five or six months of age.[17] They recommend that weaning begins with low-allergenic foods, such as root vegetables and fruit, and that grains, meat, tomatoes and pulses are introduced one at a time after a couple of weeks. There is, however, no evidence to support delaying the introduction of these foods past six months. Coeliac UK states that babies at risk (i.e. with a family history) of coeliac disease (an autoimmune disease meaning the body cannot process gluten) should not be weaned any differently from those who have no additional risk. In other words, there is no benefit in withholding wheat or gluten.[18]

Does weaning onto solids aid sleep?

Parents are often advised to 'fill up' their babies as much as possible during the day, with both milk feeds and solids, the assumption being that the more they eat during the day, the fuller they will feel at night and the less likely they will be to wake. It is also commonly suggested that they introduce solids earlier than the normal and recommended six-month point. This advice stems from the belief that night waking is always due to hunger. However, research has shown that night waking is unaffected by daytime eating.[19] Further research looking at the sleep patterns of over 700 babies aged between six and twelve months old has also disproved the theory that 'filling up' babies in the daytime improves night sleep.[20] In this study, mothers were asked to report their baby's night waking and night feeds, in addition to providing details of daytime food intake, both milk and solids. The results revealed that almost 79 per cent of six- to twelve-month-old babies still woke regularly at night and that 61 per cent of the babies still had a least one milk feed per night. There was no difference in night waking and night feeds between babies who were breastfed and babies who were formula-fed. But the most interesting finding of the research was that those babies who consumed more solid food and milk during the day didn't wake or feed any less at night than those whose consumption was lower during the day. In other words, solids and milk intake in the daytime has no impact on night waking.

Signs of weaning readiness

Although all the research seems to point to 'around six months' as the right age to begin introducing solids, this guidance does not consider individual children. The best indicator of your child's readiness for starting solids is a combination of them being close to six months of age, as well as exhibiting some behavioural and physical signs of interest. The top three signs of readiness to wean onto solids are the following:

- The baby should be able to stay in a sitting position, with support if necessary, and should be able to hold their head steady.

- The baby should be able to coordinate their eyes, hands and mouth. They should be able to look at food, grab it and put it in their mouths by themselves.

- The baby should be able to swallow their food. Babies who are not ready will often push their food back out with their tongues (something known as the tongue-thrust reflex). They will, consequently, get more food around their faces than in their mouths. At six months, most babies should have lost this reflex.

In addition to the above, the baby must show interest in solids. Some babies may display all the physical signs of readiness and have no interest in eating anything other than milk. Here, the gentle-eating way would be to stay mindful of the child's interest, as well as their abilities, and to respect that they will begin in their own time. The authoritative or responsive-feeding approach that constitutes gentle eating means that the baby is in control of what and when they eat. The hardest part as a parent is to trust in the baby, but this is also the most important part of all when it comes to introducing solids. Reminding yourself that your baby's milk intake remains the main source of nutrients throughout the whole of their first year can help you to slow down and move at your baby's pace.

To purée or not to purée?

Traditionally, solids have been introduced to a baby's diet in purée form on a spoon, the most common being fruit, vegetables and cereals. More recently, there has been a shift towards 'baby-led weaning' and giving babies 'finger foods' to self-feed, right from the very start of weaning.[21]

The key feature of baby-led weaning is that the baby is in control of eating, always. This means that purées are not given alongside finger foods and the parent doesn't ever spoon-feed the baby. Some parents will pre-load spoons with food in order that the baby can pick it up and use it to feed themselves, but if the baby chooses to ignore the spoon, the contents are discarded.

There does seem to be an increasing level of confusion surrounding baby-led weaning, and research has found that over 70 per cent of parents who believed that they were following this method were actually spoon-feeding their babies, which is completely at odds with the theory.[22]

The guiding principle behind baby-led weaning is that the baby has autonomy from the moment they start eating solids. Allowing them to control what they eat, how much and when – in line with gentle-eating principles – is said to make them better attuned to their bodily signals, enabling them to recognise and respond to their own hunger and satiety cues more readily than a baby who is being spoon-fed with purées. Research has shown that babies who were weaned using the baby-led approach were significantly more satiety-responsive and less likely to be overweight compared with those weaned using the traditional spoon-feeding method.[23]

This doesn't mean it is not possible to follow gentle-eating principles if you spoon-feed, but it is significantly harder, as you must be much more mindful of the baby's hunger and satiety cues and food preferences in order to ensure that you do not accidentally encourage them to eat more than they want or need.

Although gentle-eating principles naturally align with baby-led weaning, it does require a good level of trust on behalf of the parents (albeit a continuation of the responsive-feeding style begun in early infancy). There is no reason to not trust a baby's hunger and satiety signals once they start to eat solids, but it is not uncommon for the baby's experience with solids at the start of their weaning journey to look different from what many parents expect. Traditionally weaned babies can fairly quickly be on three 'good' meals per day and when compared to them, babies following baby-led weaning can seem as if they are not consuming enough food. Really, this goes back to my point in Chapter 1 about the erroneous belief that we should eat three regular meals per day, clearing our plates in the process. This is not a healthy practice for adults and it is not healthy for babies either.

The healthiest response that a baby can have to weaning is curiosity about food. Initially, that may not actually involve eating the food, but may just mean playing with it – babies will mush, poke, throw and stick their fingers in food, often long before they will actually eat it. But this 'playing with food' is a good sign. Babies need to learn about the sensory aspects of different foodstuffs before they begin to eat them. Mushing, poking and throwing help babies to feel confident with food. In time, a little more will make it into their mouths and some will even be swallowed. This is not a process to rush, however; it's time to sit back and let the baby take control. Research has found that babies who follow baby-led weaning achieve a similar energy intake to those weaned using traditional spoon-feeding.[24] In addition, because babies weaned following the baby-led method eat the same food as the rest of the family, rather than specially prepared baby food, right from the start of the weaning process, they are likely to be exposed to a greater range of foods and textures than those weaned traditionally, which may, in time, reduce fussiness. Research has also repeatedly shown that the only difference nutritionally between the two methods is the level of iron intake. This can be addressed, however, by following a slightly modified version of baby-led weaning developed specifically with iron in mind.[25] To reduce any negative impact on iron levels, parents are simply advised to offer an iron-rich food (such as meat or iron-fortified cereal) at each meal, alongside an energy-rich food and a fruit or vegetable. This approach allows the baby full control of their eating, but the parental input into choice of foods offered ensures that the baby's nutrient needs are more likely to be met each day.

Are there any foods to avoid?

Part of the fun of baby-led weaning is being able to offer a large range of different foods from early on. Most meals offered are those that the rest of the family are eating. There are a few foods, however, that are not appropriate for this stage:

- **Processed food, especially with added salt or sugar** Baby-led weaning often encourages more home cooking and use of fresh ingredients, which improves the parental diet too.

- **Honey** Honey contains a bacterium called *Clostridium botulinum*, the spores of which can grow and develop in a baby's digestive system, potentially causing botulism, which can be fatal.

- **Cow's milk** Regular cow's milk does not contain sufficient nutrients to replace breast milk or infant formula as a main drink until after the first year. The same is also true of almond, rice, soya and goat milks.

- **Baby rice** Aside from the rather unappealing consistency, colour and lack of taste, baby rice is highly processed and high in sugar and should, ideally, be completely avoided. It has almost no nutrients and, perhaps most alarmingly, it can contain the poison arsenic.[26] Often naturally present in the soil of rice fields, arsenic can leach into the rice itself if flooding occurs, as it commonly does. There is currently no legislation in place regarding acceptable levels of arsenic in foods. As babies are significantly smaller than adults, however, the amount of arsenic contained in rice could be much more problematic for them, and until such time as safe levels and corresponding legislation are established, it may be wise to avoid it altogether.

- **Whole grapes** Grapes present a choking hazard and should always be cut into halves or quarters. Even then, they should not be given to babies until they are experienced eaters.

In addition, parents should always be aware of the texture of the food that they are giving and avoid anything significantly crumbly that may break up into large pieces in the baby's mouth, constituting a choking hazard. Any finger foods given should be as long as the baby's fist, to enable easy handling, as well as reducing choking risk, such as a long chunk of cucumber, potato wedges or a quartered banana.

Home-made or shop-bought?

In an ideal world, none of us would eat processed foods, but it is often necessary to supplement home-made foods with commercial, ready-made ones. Research has shown that the diets of babies who were fed home-made food were more diverse than those of babies who were fed shop-bought food.[27] In addition, those fed home-made food had significantly less body fat than those fed commercial food, a trend that persisted into childhood. Furthermore, babies weaned on shop-bought, ready-prepared food consumed fewer vegetables than those weaned on home-made food. This is important to note, as further research has shown that ultimate acceptance of fruit and vegetables is linked with repeated exposure to them.[28]

The takeaway message here is to reduce the use of commercial baby foods as much as possible. If you are sharing family mealtimes and food with your baby, being mindful of reducing the amount of processed food that you eat is important. When you do need to use ready-made food, however, it should not be something to feel guilty about. Just try to keep it to a minimum and offer your baby a wide array of fresh foods as well, especially fruits and vegetables, alongside iron- and energy-rich foods.

Creating the ideal eating environment

Weaning isn't just about what the baby eats – where and how they are introduced to food are equally as important. The eating environment matters from both a physical and emotional point of view. Let's look at some of the factors that help to create the healthiest eating environment for new eaters.

- **Unhurried** Perhaps the most important thing needed to wean a baby onto solids is endless amounts of patience on your behalf. Learning to eat takes time. While you are an experienced eater, finishing your food relatively quickly, remember this is all new to your baby. Slow down. It is not unusual for a tiny amount of food to take half an hour, or even an hour to eat. Avoid hurrying your baby. If you are pushed for time, then it is better to skip a meal if your baby is not too hungry, than to give one and pressure your baby to finish quickly.

- **Distraction-free** When you offer your baby food, make sure food is the focus. Turn off the television and any tablets, put their toys away and create an environment in which your baby can focus fully on eating. Similarly, you need to focus too. Put your phone away – now isn't the time to multitask. Lastly, avoid eating on the move, especially in the earlier days of weaning.

- **Modelling** Your baby needs to learn how to eat by watching you. In fact, this happens long before weaning officially starts, but when it does begin, make sure you are the best role model possible. Take time to eat together, preferably the same food, commenting on the textures and flavours as you chew and turning the mealtime into a shared experience with conversation.

- **Relaxed** Eating should be a relaxed and enjoyable time, which is why it is so important not to hurry your baby. Before you begin the meal, take time for a few big breaths and to release any of the stresses and strains of the day. Now is the time to be calm and relaxed and not stressing over what your baby is or isn't eating. Being mindful of your own emotions and how they may impact on your baby's eating is so important.

- **Face to face** Try to arrange your eating area so that you and your baby can look into each other's eyes easily, meaning that you should, ideally, be on the same level. Many baby high chairs position the baby much too high, which means that eye contact becomes much harder if you are eating at a table together. If you are using a high chair, try to choose one that positions your baby's head at the same level as yours when you are seated at the table. Alternatively, using a booster on a chair which allows your baby to be pushed into the table is often more successful and allows them to mimic you more easily. Another good idea is to purchase a large piece of plastic table covering and sit together on the floor for meals, picnic style.

Your main goal here is to make the eating environment as calm, relaxed, pressure-free and unhurried as possible. Keep your focus on your baby, model eating and reduce distractions as much as possible. These guidelines will provide the foundations for a positive family eating environment. Working hard to produce the best environment possible right from the start will ensure you reap the rewards for many years to come.

Table manners

One of the questions I am commonly asked by parents who are weaning babies is how to encourage good table manners. Sometimes I feel that the imposition of adult eating etiquette on babies who are only just learning how to eat is a little bizarre, to say the least. I am of the opinion that this should be taken 'one step at a time'. There is plenty of time to learn table manners in the future, but for now, focusing on learning to eat is enough for your baby. In fact, some of the social rules surrounding food may inhibit the weaning process and could lead to fussy behaviour. Let's look at the top four concerns parents tend to have surrounding table manners, and consider whether they are a good match for babies who are learning how to eat.

Introducing cutlery

When babies begin to eat solid food themselves they will pick it up with their hands. This is in sharp contrast to adults who have been taught that it is rude to eat with your hands and who use a knife, fork or spoon instead. I think we must differentiate here between the abilities of adults, with their mature dexterity and manual control and well-practised eating skills, and those of babies who have barely learned to grasp something, bring it to their mouths and suck and chew on it. In time, with more control and experience, babies will begin to use cutlery of their own accord because they will copy adults. This is one of the reasons why it is so important to eat with babies, so that they can observe how we do it. It is a good idea to give them cutlery to play with from very early on, but you shouldn't expect them to eat reliably with it until well into the toddler years and even beyond.

Playing with food

As adults, we know it is rude to 'play with our food'. Babies, on the other hand, need to do this. They need to squish it, squash it, mush it, roll it, smear it and wipe it. And although this may seem like 'naughty' behaviour at first glance, it is actually an essential part of learning to eat. The sensory experience of eating, via touch, is almost as important as that of taste. Babies need to understand the texture and properties of different foods and 'playing with it' is how they do it. If this sensory learning is prohibited, or if the baby is made to be fearful of mess, perhaps through frequent cleaning by parents, they may grow to be a fussier eater as a result.

Throwing food

Throwing food is often an extension of play. It may also happen if the baby's satiety signals are missed or ignored. If the baby is full, but unable to indicate verbally to an adult that they have finished eating, throwing food is a pretty successful way to get attention and divert it away from eating. If this is the cause, take it as a sign that you need to be more mindful about your baby's hunger and satiety cues and learn to accept and respect them, no matter what you think about the amount of food they have consumed.

Another reason why babies will often throw food from a high chair is due to something called a trajectory schema. A schema is a learning and thought process and a stage of development that teaches children about the way the world works. The trajectory schema teaches the baby about movement, mass and direction. Babies will often throw items to observe their trajectory – for instance, food thrown from their high chair or water thrown into the air. This is a normal stage of development and will pass naturally. Until it does, you may consider moving your child onto a big mat on the floor, or placing less food out for them to throw from the high chair, cleaning up any that is thrown in a very calm and matter-of-fact way.

Sitting at the table until everybody has finished

Although eating together as a family is one of the best ways to raise a happy and healthy eater, the adult expectation of every-one sitting quietly at the table until the last person has finished is an unrealistic one for babies. If a baby has finished eating and is not content to continue sitting at the table, there is no benefit in trying to force them to stay there. Young children do not have the same impulse control as adults, and babies will find it impossible to sit quietly at the table when they no longer have any interest in eating. Respecting this and allowing them to play or leave the table is not impolite. It is understanding and accept-ing of their neurological capabilities. There are many years ahead in which to teach your baby to sit quietly at the table once they have finished eating, but now is not the time. Even worse, trying to encourage them to continue eating because others are still doing so teaches them to ignore their satiety signals and overeat.

We must remember that babies are not adults and, as such, we shouldn't expect them to behave like us at mealtimes. The best way to encourage babies to develop good table manners is to model them ourselves. Be mindful of how you eat: do you always demonstrate the table manners you would like your child to learn?

Are solids more important than milk?

The term 'weaning' is a misleading one because it implies that the introduction of solids into the baby's diet means that they will wean from milk and no longer consume it. In fact, weaning doesn't mean stopping milk at all. Milk remains the most important part of a baby's diet for at least the first twelve months. We have already seen, earlier in this chapter, just how many of the required nutrients are gained from milk.

For the first year of the baby's life, solid foods should be supplementary to milk, not a replacement. Viewing solids as complementing milk helps us to be more realistic about the amount of food a baby needs to eat. Similarly, while the amount of milk consumed each day gradually falls between six and twelve months, as solid food is introduced, the baby will usually still consume more milk than anything else. If babies are slow to take to solids, as many are, the common advice is to cut back on the milk to increase hunger. But this advice is naive, as most of the solid foods consumed by the baby will contain fewer nutrients and fewer calories than milk. Compare, for instance, half a stick of carrot and a cup of milk – the milk clearly has far more of what the baby needs. The ideal goal should be to work at the baby's pace and keep introducing new foods, repeatedly, if they have been discarded before, and stay mindful of the iron content, while allowing the baby to consume as much milk as they need.

Some babies simply take longer to enjoy solids than others. My daughter had little interest in solids until she was ten months old, and even then, she was nearer to twelve or thirteen months by the time she really took to them. Now, ten years on, my 'milk monster' eats a varied diet, is a healthy weight and has a great relationship with food.

Remember, solids are complementary to milk, not a replacement for it.

Common worries when starting solids

I think it is worth spending a little time looking at a few specific concerns held by many parents of older babies.

Choking on food

Many parents are anxious about the possibility of their baby choking when they are eating solids, particularly finger foods. While there is a chance that this may happen, the risk is very small. In fact, much of what parents believe is choking is actually gagging. Whereas choking presents a medical emergency, gagging is an entirely normal and healthy physiological response. Differentiating between the two is therefore important:

Gagging	Choking
Common	Uncommon
No risk posed to baby	Dangerous
Caused by food reaching farther down the back of the throat, triggering the gag reflex to move it forward	Caused by food entering the upper airway and blocking the baby's air flow
Loud	Silent
No intervention required – the baby will cough and gag the food back up independently	Immediate intervention required

Gagging is common, especially when weaning with finger foods. Trusting your baby to cough up the food and not intervening is the best response, although witnessing it for the first time can be distressing. If your baby is making a loud noise, then that's a good sign. Choking, on the other hand, is virtually silent as the food is blocking the baby's airway and ability to breathe. The recommended response to choking is to ask somebody to call the emergency services, while you first check to see if you can easily remove the object, being careful not to lodge it farther in. If you are unable to remove it, then you should turn the baby over your arm and give them five sharp back blows between their shoulder blades with the heel of your hand to dislodge the object. If you are alone with your baby, call the emergency services after working on them for two minutes. This process is significantly easier to understand and remember if you learn it direct from a paediatric first-aid course. Attending a course gives you a level of confidence that you just don't get from watching a video or reading a book. I attended a course a few months before my daughter was born, never expecting to use what I had learned. Less than a year later I put it into practice when she began choking one day having put a small piece of a toy belonging to one of her brothers in her mouth. My instinct immediately took over and I used what I had learned from the course. I could not see the object, so I turned her over and gave her five sharp back blows, while yelling for my husband to call 999. Several more back blows later, and with an ambulance on the way, the object finally dislodged and she let out a loud cry. I will never forget how wonderful that cry was after a minute of silence with her turning blue. I have counted my blessings for my decision to attend the first-aid course many times. I'm not sure what would have happened otherwise; it's not something I want to think about. My daughter was a big 'gagger' when weaning, but the difference between the loud and frequent normal physiological gagging, often accompanied by a red face, and the silent choking while her face turned blue was dramatic. Although choking and gagging are commonly mixed up, they couldn't be more different.

Research has found that while babies who are weaned using a baby-led approach gag more than those who are weaned using traditional spoon-feeding with purées, there is no difference in the level of choking.[29]

Only eating carbohydrates and sweet foods

Babies naturally prefer savoury and sweet flavours, while they naturally dislike bitter and sour tastes. It is commonly theorised that these tastes are a result of a biological drive towards high energy and high protein, to aid growth, and an aversion to foods that may be toxic and poisonous, thus presenting a risk to life. Most babies therefore prefer to eat carbohydrates, such as bread-based products, and sweet foods, such as apples, pears and bananas.[30] Repeated exposure to previously rejected foods, alongside good modelling from parents, will ultimately lead to a more adventurous palate. In the meantime, remember that milk still offers a large proportion of the baby's nutritional needs.

Only eating dry foods

Many babies struggle with 'slimy food' and will only eat foods such as breadsticks and crackers. Weaning is a learning process and learning takes time. Slimy food and even food with sauce can be alarming to babies as it does not have a texture that they have come across before. They are used to liquids and to putting all manner of hard and dry objects (albeit not food) in their mouths before weaning begins, such as teething toys, dummies and the like. Slimy is something new. The key here is to help the baby to feel more at ease with the texture through play. Again, they are used to playing with liquids, such as water in the bath, and with hard, dry objects (almost all their toys), but they are not used to anything in between. Setting up messy play with jelly, cheap hair gel and tapioca and encouraging them to stick their hands into the slimy mixtures, while you make positive comments, will help to normalise the texture and, ultimately, lead to their acceptance of eating foods with that consistency.

Solids regression

Regressions with weaning are common. Just as you think you have turned a corner, your baby will get sick or start teething and their interest in eating will disappear. This is normal. We often don't feel like eating if we are ill, in pain or convalescing. In addition, it is common for babies to increase their milk intake in times of illness or pain, as they strongly equate breast- or bottle-feeding with comfort and calm. Some babies can also become slightly phobic about eating solids if they link it with vomiting. If they have previously had a vomiting bug or reflux, and remember the distress of vomiting up solid food, they may avoid eating it once they are better. The answer here is patience and time. Trust that your baby will develop an interest in eating solids again; don't pressure them. Keep offering, but allow them to leave the food untouched, while saying, 'It's OK, you don't want to eat today', as you clear it away. Modelling here is as important as ever. By eating with your baby, you show them that it can be a positive and happy experience and nothing to fear.

Eating too much

While most concerns about eating in the early months, or indeed the early years, focus on fussy eating and food refusal, some parents have the opposite worry. Some babies can seem to like food a little too much. Should you be concerned if your baby always wants to eat? Providing your baby is otherwise healthy, you are not offering overly fatty, sugary or processed food and you are following his hunger and satiety cues carefully, you can relax. Some babies prefer eating solids to milk and often, when their solids intake increases dramatically, their milk intake declines, which will even out their energy intake. Some babies seem to need a lot of solids and a lot of milk. Often, these are the 'busy babies' – busy growing and busy moving. Once again, their energy intake is usually a good match for their energy expenditure. If you are certain that you are not encouraging emotional eating, or that they are eating when they are not hungry, the ethos of gentle eating is clear: trust your baby and respect that they know what they need.

When should you wean off milk?

There really is no specific age to wean your baby off milk. Again, being led by them is usually best. If you are formula-feeding, you should continue to give formula milk, preferably 'first milk', until your baby is twelve months old, after which you can switch to regular cow's milk. It is a good idea to slowly replace your baby's bottles with a beaker when possible and begin to wean from bottles. Research has shown that the number of milk feeds given by bottle is positively correlated with the chance of the baby being overweight.[31] The bottles your baby would usually have when they are awake is the easiest place to begin, leaving bottles at bedtime and naptime till last, as they are usually harder to wean if the baby takes comfort from them.

When should you stop breastfeeding?

The media and Western society in general seem to believe that breastfeeding should stop around the time that a baby cuts his or her first teeth. For most babies, this is somewhere around six to twelve months of age. After this, many feel that breastfeeding no longer benefits the child, but rather, is something that the mother does to try to prove a point or keep her baby younger for longer. Society feels that in fulfilling their own needs these mothers may psychologically harm their children, stifling their independence. Many people state that they find it 'odd' and would feel deeply uncomfortable if they saw an older child breastfeeding. In other countries around the world, however, it is completely normal to breastfeed to age three and beyond, and in these societies they feel that we, in the West, are 'odd'.

Most mothers who breastfeed an older child don't set out with the intention to continue until a certain age, although many do plan on letting the weaning be dictated by their child's needs and not their own. Time passes quickly and you don't notice your baby growing, until suddenly you realise that they are now three or four years old and breastfeeding, that normal part of everyday life, is continuing. This is certainly the position I found myself in when my daughter self-weaned from breastfeeding just shy of her fifth birthday. I must admit I was one of the people who found 'natural-term breastfeeding' odd before I did it myself. When I was doing it, though, it was just a part of everyday life and felt totally natural and – importantly – normal! I certainly couldn't have forced my daughter to carry on breastfeeding against her will. The whole process was totally led by her.

Breastfeeding is not only about nutrition. It is also a wonderful comfort to a child. Many natural-term breast feeders comment on how breastfeeding sees them through numerous illnesses, accidents and teething easily. Natural-term breastfeeding (or extended, as it is sometimes called) is not about a mother's need to 'keep her child a baby', but about meeting that child's needs. If the child is not ready to wean from the breast, the most responsive parenting approach would be to not force it. We frequently hear about the benefits of initiating breastfeeding, yet little is said about how these benefits continue well beyond infancy. In the UK, only 3 per cent of babies are exclusively breastfed at five months of age, despite the World Health Organization recommending that 'babies are breastfed from birth until two years and then as long as mutually desired'. Indeed, in many countries experts estimate that the natural age for weaning is somewhere around three or four years of age. Breastfeeding past infancy is the norm for our species and yet, ironically, it is often seen as something unnatural and abnormal.

Breastfeeding past infancy has significant health benefits for children. Breast milk is still a major source of nutrition well into the toddler years. Natural-term breastfeeding has health benefits for mothers too, with the increased length of breastfeeding protecting against varying forms of cancer and osteoporosis. If possible, the healthiest start for your baby is to allow them to self-wean from the breast, when they are ready, but what happens if you can't, or don't want to wait that long? Let's look at the gentlest way to wean from breastfeeding next.

Gentle weaning from breastfeeding

If you have reached a point where you need or really want to wean your baby from breastfeeding, then following a slow, step-by-step plan makes the experience gentler and easier for both of you. My best advice would be to choose a time to begin the weaning when everything else in your life is constant. Steer clear of the run-up to holidays, moving house, starting day care, the birth of a new sibling and any other periods of change. Pick a time when your baby is well and happy, avoiding periods of illness and teething.

Your first step is to night-wean all feeds, bar the feeding to sleep. This means that whenever your baby wakes in the night, you would aim to settle them back to sleep with cuddles and offering water. This can often be easier if you have another adult to help, because if Mum tries to do the settling, the baby can often get very upset and confused due to the presence of her breasts. Night weaning should ideally be taken slowly, working on settling without feeding, one wake at a time, and ensuring that the baby is always being comforted and 'in arms', not left to cry alone. I generally don't recommend night weaning before nine months as an absolute minimum, but ideally twelve months, because before this babies often do need the nutrition of milk in the night and the weaning is likely to be stressful for all involved. If you do try to night-wean before this point, you should offer a bottle or cup of milk in place of water.

Once the baby is reliably night weaned, the next step is to wean from all feeds in the day that are not related to naptimes – so the first morning feed and all feeds in between naps. In place of these, offer water or milk from a cup or bottle. Once the day-time 'waking feeds' are weaned, then the next step is to wean from the feeding to sleep for naptimes. Here, once again, offer a cup or bottle of milk and lots of comfort and cuddles. Finally, the last feed to wean is the bedtime one. This is often by far the hardest to drop in my opinion as it is usually the one babies need the most. I would therefore consider if it is possible to retain it for a while longer – many parents do find that it is easier to keep this one feed until the baby naturally outgrows it. If you cannot, or don't want to keep the bedtime feed, then once again, you are looking at offering milk from a bottle or cup and lots of comfort, rocking, singing, patting, stroking and so on. It is common for bedtimes to regress when you are no longer feeding to sleep and it may be significantly harder to get your baby to sleep without the bedtime breastfeed. If you really do need, or want, to stop all feeding, then empathising with your baby, supporting them while they cry and staying consistent is the key.

Questions from parents

Throughout the remainder of this book I have included some questions in each chapter from parents who are struggling with some aspect of eating. This chapter features questions from three parents, each at a different point on the weaning journey. I hope you'll find their questions and my responses useful.

Q. *My partner and I recently became first-time parents to our son, who is now four months. My son is currently* *exclusively breastfed and he has an expressed bottle once a week. We are looking to start the weaning process when he hits six months old. We are just starting to consider the best methods of weaning, but it is a bit of a minefield, so any advice or guidance would be appreciated. My main questions are: where do we start? What foods are best? And what about portion sizes? As first-time parents, we are pretty clueless.*

A. It is recommended to begin weaning at around six months of age, although the actual age of readiness – both physiological and psychological – is different for each baby. There is nothing magical that happens on the day of your baby's first half birthday – he may be ready to start a few weeks earlier or a few weeks later, so the key is being led by him. Look out for him being interested in eating food, able to grasp it and bring it up to his mouth himself and ultimately to swallow the food, not just push it out of his mouth again. He should also be able to sit upright, with a little support, if necessary.

The more you can leave the weaning process up to your son, the better. I would suggest following baby-led weaning, offering finger foods only and avoiding all spoon-feeding, unless he uses the spoon to feed himself. This method means that your son has as much control as possible over the process and is more likely to establish a good relationship with food. I would start by offering him small amounts of the food that you are eating yourself, providing that it is home-cooked and unprocessed. Avoid anything with added salt and sugar and steer clear of honey too until after his first birthday. Make sure that you offer him food in strips and chunks that are easy for him to hold, around the same length as his fist. Good 'first foods' are soft vegetables (lightly cooked carrot batons, jacket potato wedges, broccoli florets and fingers of parsnip), fruits (lightly stewed apple slices, bananas, pear slices and avocado strips), cheese sticks, hard-boiled or scrambled egg, chunks of cooked meat (chicken, beef, ham) and toast fingers. Try to aim for each meal to contain one food that is rich in iron (for instance, meat), one that is rich in energy (for instance, cheese) and one that is eaten more readily (often carbohydrates). Offer him food when you eat; the more he can watch you eat and copy you, the easier weaning will be.

Don't worry about the amount he eats. In the early days, weaning is more about introducing him to the concept of eating solid food than about the quantity consumed. He is likely to squish, smear and throw the food, which is normal, and actually playing with the food is also part of the learning process, as it helps him to understand the different sensory properties of food. In terms of nutrition, he will get most of what he needs from milk for several more months – view the solids as complementary to his milk, not a replacement for it. He is unlikely to eat 'three full meals' a day until sometime after his first birthday. This is normal too. Don't panic when he refuses certain foods, especially vegetables. Just keep re-offering food he has previously refused – it can take hundreds of exposures before he eats certain things, particularly vegetables. Most of all, though, try to trust that he will eat if he is hungry; don't force him to eat more than he wants and don't try to hurry him along. Similarly, if he wants more food, even though you think he has already eaten a lot, trust that he knows his body's needs better than you. Weaning really is all about trust: you trusting your baby's needs and your baby learning to trust his own body's signals.

Q. *My daughter is eight months old, and we started baby-led weaning two months ago. Up until that point she was exclusively breastfed, and I am continuing to breastfeed alongside solids. She has never had milk (breast or formula)* *from a bottle. She is strong-willed and refuses to be fed – if anyone tries, she purses her lips, moves her head from side to side and pushes their hand away. I am giving her three meals a day, but she is consuming little . . . it is so frustrating!*

For breakfast, I offer porridge (on a preloaded spoon, or cooled and in thick fingers), Weetabix, fruit, toast, eggs, eggy bread; for lunch, fruit, vegetables, muffins, cheese, puff-pastry wheels, etc.; and for dinner, whatever my husband and I are eating (if it's baby friendly, obviously). Sometimes she will have a little, but, mostly, she pushes the food around, mushes it up and throws it on the floor. She will eat rice cakes and pitta breads, and sometimes some fruit such as mango, but that isn't a balanced, nutritious diet! Also, she doesn't really drink any water. I offer it to her from a free-flow cup and a doidy cup [a special open-top cup designed for babies], but she tends to push both away. I have given her the free-flow cup to drink from herself, but she flings it around and barely drinks from it. She won't let me help her to drink either. I am giving her vitamin D drops.

I can't help but worry that she's not getting the nutrients she needs, particularly iron, and that she won't get the hang of eating. It's also so disheartening spending lots of time preparing, 'eating' and cleaning up from meals when she barely eats anything, and so much ends up on the floor and in the bin. Should I be worried? Is there a different approach I can try?

A. Your daughter sounds perfectly normal to me. Her eating is exactly what I would expect from a baby who has only been eating solids for a couple of months. Allowing her to control her own eating – both the physical aspect of putting food into her mouth and respecting her own hunger and satiety cues – will afford her the very best start to her relationship with food. At this age, she is getting most of the nutrients that she needs from milk, as well as from the vitamin D supplement that you are giving her. The only nutrient that she may be low on currently is iron, as her iron stores from birth will be depleting and she is not eating much iron-rich solid food. That said, she will absorb around 50 per cent of the iron contained in breast milk, compared to around 10 per cent of that in in other foods (even those that are iron-rich), so although levels of iron in breast milk are low, the fact that it is so much better absorbed negates some of the issue. I would suggest that you offer your daughter something containing iron with each meal, and alongside this I would give her something you know she will eat and a new or previously refused food.

In terms of the amount she eats, and what she refuses, you should really try to not worry about this. It is normal for babies to refuse more than they eat initially. Your daughter is learning about her own likes and dislikes, as well as her own hunger and satiety cues. Milk is still her main source of nutrients, not food, and you should view solids as complementary to her milk diet, not a replacement for it. In time, she will begin to consume more and her tastes will ever so gradually widen. You must learn to trust that she knows when she is hungry and when she is full. Research shows that babies who are weaned using baby-led weaning consume the same amount of energy, calorie-wise, as those weaned using traditional spoon-feeding, but they do grow to have a healthier relationship with food and fewer weight problems. I understand you are questioning your approach right now, but you really have chosen the healthiest route for your daughter.

Next, I understand your daughter is squishing, mushing and throwing food – probably more than she is eating. This too is normal and actually it's quite necessary! Weaning also involves learning about the textures and sensory properties of foods and wanting to understand them more. This 'playing' with food has been shown to reduce fussiness and picky eating and is not something that should be discouraged. In fact, I would encourage it more. If you have any food that is past its best, think about ways that you could use it to allow your daughter more sensory food play. Also, don't be in a rush to clean your daughter up; wiping away the 'mess' can indicate to her that food is 'yucky' and you may inadvertently turn her off eating foods with certain textures, creating sensory-based fussiness. Once your daughter is comfortable with the new sensory properties of food, she will begin to taste and then, finally, swallow it in her own time. Here, the more you can eat with her, sitting together at the table eating the same foods at the same time, the more she will mimic you and, ultimately, consume more of the food you offer her. I would say most babies get the hang of what you may call 'proper eating' using a baby-led approach by around ten to twelve months of age. Before this it really is much more about learning than nutrition.

Finally, I wouldn't be concerned by your daughter's refusal of water. Breast milk provides all the liquids she needs. I would keep offering water with each meal, trying a few different cups – ones with straws are usually quite popular – but I wouldn't make a big fuss over it. Just leave it alongside her and say, 'Here's your water'. Again, in time, she will drink it – especially if you model drinking your own cup of water at the same time.

Q. *My little girl is twelve months old and I'd like to gently wean her off breastfeeding by fourteen months at the latest. My reason for weaning is that she will only be fed to sleep. She wakes frequently and the lack of sleep is taking its toll. I recently had bad flu and pleurisy and still had to do all the nights, so couldn't really rest. I want to be able to share night duties with my husband. Also, I'm three stone overweight and I'd like to get my body back. We tried night weaning for* *three nights with my husband when he was off work. It worked by night three, and she slept great, but it didn't last and whenever I go in she just wants to breastfeed. We tried again this weekend and she just wouldn't settle for my husband. I can't handle it when she cries. Please help me to gently wean my boob monster!*

A. The gentlest way to end the breastfeeding relationship is to allow the child to lead the way and self-wean. However, I can appreciate that you are ready to end breastfeeding sooner than this. I think it is possible to wean in a way that is kind to your daughter, but I am concerned that you won't get the result that you hope for. While weaning from breastfeeding will mean that others can help to put your daughter to sleep in the evening, giving you a break, it can make getting her to sleep very hard. You may find that bedtimes are much more difficult when you can no longer feed to sleep; similarly, night weaning doesn't always solve night waking, and sometimes it can make it worse. Also, you may not find weight loss any easier when you are no longer breastfeeding. In fact, the extra calories that you are burning now by breastfeeding may actually mean that you put on weight when you stop. I am aware that so far, my reply sounds very negative, and I am not trying to put you off ending breastfeeding. Rather, I would like you to go into it fully informed with reasonable expectations, and I'm not sure whether your expectations of what life will be like when you are no longer breastfeeding are completely realistic at the moment.

If you decide that you do definitely want to go ahead, my recommendation is to wean from feeds in the following order:

1. Night feeds
2. Daytime feeds that are not immediately before a nap

3. Daytime feeds that are immediately before a nap
4. The bedtime feed

You made a good start by beginning with the night feeds and by involving your husband, but it sounds as if your daughter wasn't quite ready when you tried. I would try again by working with one feed at a time (so Dad only settles her once in the night and you breastfeed the other wakes), or by limiting the amount of time Dad attempts to settle at each wake. For instance, he might attempt to settle for five or ten minutes maximum and then you breastfeed. You can stretch the time Dad comforts a little every day until, ultimately, he is comforting for long enough to get your daughter back to sleep without a feed. Once all night feeds have gone, I would take a break for a few days and then focus on the daytime feeds that are not near to naptimes (feeding to sleep). Here, follow similar principles to the night feeds. Once most of the daytime feeds have gone, then I would work on settling her for naps without feeding. Ultimately, you will be left with the bedtime feed. This is by far the hardest feed to lose as usually it is the one that is most important to the child. Breastfeeding at bedtime not only calms and provides nutrition, but the milk also contains chemicals that aid sleep. I would therefore recommend that you consider keeping just the bedtime feed for a few months. If you are certain that you want to drop all feeds, however, then I'm afraid you will struggle to get rid of the bedtime feed. You should look to cuddle, rock, stroke, pat your daughter, offer her milk or water from a cup or bottle and consider giving her a dummy. She will likely cry a fair amount and bedtime will probably take much longer, so be prepared for this. Focus on staying calm, remind yourself that it's OK that she's upset and, most importantly of all, make sure she is always 'in arms' while she cries. The worst is usually over within the first week, although it may take several months until bedtimes become easier again – but at least you won't be doing it alone, as now others will be able to help!

The first few months of eating solids is an important time to practise responsive feeding. Understanding that weaning is not just about nutrition, but also learning and discovery, helps to take some of the pressure off you and your baby. Viewing solids as complementary to, not a replacement for, their main source of nutrition – namely milk – can often enable parents to relax and enjoy the process a little more. Allowing your baby to take control of the process and demonstrating that you trust him to do so, even during the times when not everything is going to plan, sends a strong message to him, and one that will stay with him for years to come. It is a message of belief, respect and empowerment that will help to instil gentle-eating principles for life.

Chapter 5

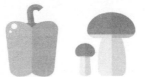

Toddler and Preschooler Eating – One to Four Years

The age group that is most synonymous with eating woes is surely the toddler/preschooler years. Picky eating almost always tops the list here, with some children taking it to extremes, barely eating anything at all and causing endless anxiety for their parents. Some, on the other hand, never seem to stop eating, although often their diet seems to consist solely of beige foods. In this chapter, we will investigate what makes these years the hardest for so many parents. We will ask why picky eating is so common, especially after a good start in babyhood, and consider how you can gently steer your child towards healthy eating habits in the future.

Let's start with a quick reminder of the gentle-eating principles. Gentle eating is:

- mindful

- empowering

- respectful

- authoritative.

In the toddler years, this means being mindful, by allowing your child to have as much control as possible over their eating, especially when it comes to their hunger and satiety levels, and also respecting their personal taste preferences, something we will discuss later in this chapter. The aim of gentle eating in toddlerhood is to empower children to become confident and relaxed eaters. Taking an authoritative approach to eating during the toddler years can help to reduce many of the eating issues that children and parents often struggle with later on, such as bingeing and dieting.

Toddlerhood is arguably the most challenging developmental period eating-wise. That's why this chapter focuses almost solely on the common problems and how to cope with them. Whether you are reading this in advance of the toddler years, or you have a toddler who doesn't seem to have any issues with eating, gentle-eating principles still very much apply and I would recommend reading this chapter in order to be as informed and mindful as possible.

When 'good-eater' babies become 'picky-eater' toddlers

Towards the end of babyhood, parents can often feel confident about their child's eating. After any initial bumps in the weaning road, babies may take to eating solids with gusto. It is common for parents to feel proud about their 'good eater' – the baby with a good appetite who eats a large variety of food, especially those considered to be healthy. By the time he had had his first birthday, my eldest son was one of those 'good eaters'. He would eat practically anything I put in front of him. I remember feeling particularly proud one evening when he ate a whole bowl of sardines, sweet potato and spinach for dinner. Cooking for him was a joy. I would spend hours steaming organic vegetables that we had delivered as part of a box scheme from a local farm, and he would reward me with gummy smiles of appreciation. I felt like a 'good mum' and thought I had the whole eating thing sorted. I didn't understand why so many parents complained about their child's eating. In fact, I believed that they had brought the problems upon themselves, by not offering their child a good range of different tastes and textures and instead pandering to their children. Oh, how wrong I was.

Around two months after his first birthday, my 'good-eater' son pretty much stopped eating. Foods he had previously wolfed down were left untouched, met with grimaces and tears. My easy baby with the good appetite was replaced with a tricky toddler who would only eat food if it was white, beige, yellow or brown and dry (sauces were pushed away with disgust), and who acted as if he was being poisoned if anything green came within arm's length. His appetite seemed to shrink in reverse correlation with his growth: the bigger he got, the less he would eat. My baby with the hearty appetite and rolls of comforting fat was replaced by a skinny little boy with the appetite of a sparrow. I no longer felt like such a good mum. In fact, I felt like a complete failure. Each day I felt as if I was failing my son – failing to keep him healthy, failing to provide him with the nutrients he needed to grow big and healthy. Days out with friends, whose toddlers ate, became torture. Lunchtime would come, and while their children ate whatever was put in front of them, my son would push a few raisins and a breadstick around his plate. The other mothers would try to placate me: 'Oh, I'm sure he'll be fine, don't worry', but the more I tried not to worry, the more anxious and obsessed with his eating I became. I started to believe that he was doing it on purpose. I begged him to eat, scolded him to eat, bribed and rewarded him to eat. I spent hours trying to hide vegetables in food. I bought special cutlery with aeroplanes on it and pretended to fly the spoon into his mouth. But nothing worked. I only wish I had known then what I know now. It would have saved me and perhaps more importantly, my son, months of anguish and stress.

You see, my son was entirely normal. Now, he is a big, burly teenager, scraping six feet tall. He eats like a horse – even green foods and foods with sauces! So what did I do to produce this miraculous change in eating habits? How did I turn my non-eating toddler into a healthy teen with a voracious appetite? In truth, I didn't do anything. In fact, it was when I stopped trying to change him – when I relaxed and accepted his eating – that the transformation happened. The most powerful thing I did was to educate myself about eating in early childhood. Once I understood his eating, or rather lack of it, I was able to relax.

The causes of picky eating

The most compelling thing I learned about childhood eating as a parent was that picky eating is normal. By normal, I mean there are genuine physiological reasons why it exists and these are often rooted in keeping the child safe. The relief I felt when I understood that the very behaviour I thought was hurting my son was actually protecting him was immense. I hope I can share some of that relief with you in this section, as I outline some the top causes of picky eating.

Neophobia

Neophobia is used to describe an irrational fear or dislike of anything unfamiliar or new. In the case of eating, it refers to the instant dislike children – particularly toddlers and pre-schoolers – take to any new foods, even without tasting them. Neophobia is the norm, rather than the exception to the rule, in young children. While it may be incredibly frustrating for parents, especially after they have lovingly prepared a meal to introduce their child to a new taste or ingredient, it is actually important to the child's survival. Think back to a time before food regulation, sanitised food shopping and ingredients labels – a time when we would have lived 'in the wild', when we would have hunted or gathered our food ourselves. Hungry children would have foraged for food and eaten what they found. So from an evolutionary perspective, neophobia would have kept young children safe. By avoiding foods that they had not previously eaten, children would avoid any potential toxins found in the new foods. When young children stick to eating only what they know, they demonstrate an important evolutionary throwback. Although the new foods offered by parents today may be completely safe, the child's instinctive drive to refuse them remains unchanged from the one that protected children hundreds, if not thousands, of years ago.

Research has shown that most children develop a degree of food neophobia when they turn two years old.[1] Predominantly, this means that the toddler will stop accepting new foods that are offered to them, although many also begin to refuse foods that they previously ate. Children are significantly more unlikely to eat foods at two years of age that they previously ate as babies.[2] This refusal may be because they don't remember eating the food before or it may be that they associate the food with a negative experience. Sometimes there is no obvious reason for the refusal, but parents can take heart from the fact that this pattern is very common and very normal and usually entirely temporary (albeit not as temporary as parents would like).

Genetics

Another way in which nature protects young children from being accidentally poisoned is to make toxic foods unpalatable. From birth, we favour sweet and savoury tastes and tend to dislike sour and bitter ones. This is no surprise when you realise that most poisonous substances have a bitter taste. Our innate taste preferences help to keep us safe and prevent us from accidentally ingesting foods that could endanger our lives, in a similar way to food neophobia.[3] The only slight flaw in nature's plan is that there is a class of compounds contained in some foods, known as glucosinolates, which are bitter tasting and can sometimes be toxic, but not always. Safe glucosinolates naturally occur in certain fruits and vegetables, such as broccoli, cabbage, kale and Brussels sprouts and many other green vegetables – the very same vegetables that most toddlers and preschoolers dislike so much. Quite simply, there is a very real physiological reason why children don't 'eat their greens'; they are genetically pre-programmed not to, in order to stay alive!

All children have a natural aversion to bitter tastes, but some find them much harder to tolerate than others. In fact, some adults struggle significantly with bitter-tasting food too. Perhaps you do? Or perhaps you know an adult who does? Again, the reason is genetic and entirely normal, as we discussed earlier (see page 18).

The bitter compound phenylthiocarbamide (or PTC for short) is detected by a specific taste receptor governed by the TAS2R28 gene. PTC sensitivity is variable, depending on each individual's specific gene encoding, meaning that the ability to detect PTC, or bitterness, is different for everyone. Some people will be sensitive to very small amounts of PTC and have a low tolerance level for bitter tastes as a result, while others will have very low sensitivity and can therefore tolerate very high levels of bitterness. Still others will not be able to detect PTC at all. The ability to taste PTC is closely linked to that for detecting other bitter substances found in nature, such as glucosinolates. Those who are 'strong tasters', or more commonly dubbed 'super tasters' by the media, are far more sensitive to bitter tastes than others. Strong tasters make up around a quarter of the population (both adult and child). Research has also found that children with high PTC sensitivity are significantly more sensitive to bitter tastes than adults with high PTC sensitivity.[4] Or, in other words, children experience stronger tastes, particularly bitter ones, more than adults because our sense of taste fades with age. So there is hope that they will venture into consuming them as they grow older and their sensitivity to bitterness fades.

There are likely other genetic factors governing food fussiness too, not just related to bitterness perception. Research looking at the eating habits of three-year-old twins has shown a significant genetic impact on food fussiness and eating behaviours.[5] Similarly, children who are picky eaters tend to have parents who are picky eaters, especially when considering vegetable intake.[6] While there is clearly a psychological effect when it comes to the impact of modelling and learned behaviour, there is also undoubtedly an underlying genetic influence. Too often, we expect our children to eat foods that we don't like very much ourselves, when perhaps we would be better off considering whether they have inherited the same trait responsible for our own dislikes.

Autonomy struggles

There are only three aspects of their lives that toddlers and preschoolers can control: sleeping, toileting and eating. Parents may control almost everything in a child's life, but they cannot make a child sleep, go to the toilet or chew and swallow food. These things are solely the domain of the child. Why does this matter? Because if a child is struggling with autonomy over their own life, then eating is one of the areas that can become problematic. If they feel suffocated by their schedule, with too many boundaries, too little opportunity for free and independent play and not enough scope for child-led activities, they often seek to gain the control that they want via their eating. Picky eating may sometimes have its roots in a totally different aspect of the child's life, although there is often a lack of autonomy felt around actual eating too.

A good example here is to think about what you ate yesterday. Think about each particular item you ate: who chose it? Who chose how you ate it, when you ate it, the temperature it was served at? What about where you ate it and the portion size? Who decided when you had had enough? Or if you had more? The chances are that your answer to all of these questions was 'Me'. Now consider the same questions, only this time in relation to your child. We may think that we are giving children control over their eating, but we're not; or not much, anyway. Parents often say to me, 'But I always give my child a choice – I ask if they want pasta or fish, a cheese or a ham sandwich, cornflakes or porridge . . . ' In response, I always ask the parents to imagine themselves in a restaurant. They are given a menu to choose from and expect to see perhaps ten different options for each course, maybe more. Upon opening the menu, however, they find only two choices: chicken done one way or a vegetarian lasagne. I then ask them, what would they think of that menu?

Would they consider it a good one? Or would they exclaim, 'Wow, what a poor choice! Only two different options?' Now ask yourself again if you are really giving your child a good choice when you let them choose between two different options to eat? Of course, you can't prepare a restaurant-worthy menu every day, but getting your child involved in selecting food when you purchase it, offering at least three different options at each meal and allowing the child to select how much of each meal component they would like on their plate when it comes to serving provides a much better level of choice and control than simply, 'Do you want this or that?'

We don't just take away control over what a child eats, though, we also control how they eat it (fingers or cutlery, but only with specific foods: sometimes fingers are OK, sometimes they're not); where they eat it (at the table); what time they eat it (lunchtime is at twelve o'clock, dinner is at five o'clock); the types of food they eat at specific times (cereal for breakfast, sandwiches for lunch – never the other way round); the order they eat the food in (dessert always comes after dinner, not before); the temperature it's served at ('Eat your food quickly, before it gets cold'); and what constitutes an acceptable blend of foods ('No, you can't have fish fingers with custard, don't be silly'). We also tend to override our children's hunger and satiety ('You can't be hungry – you only just ate dinner' or 'You can't be full up, you've barely eaten anything all day'), as well as not truly respecting their taste preferences ('Oh, it's lovely – how can you say you don't like it? Just eat a bit more'). Research has shown that the more controlling a parent is about their child's eating, the fussier the child will become.[7] Even those who feel they are giving their child as much control as possible over their eating most likely aren't. Giving more control back to the child is an important consideration when trying to improve picky eating.

Sensory struggles

When we think about toddlers and preschoolers refusing certain foods, we generally think it's because they don't like the taste. While this is undoubtedly true, particularly for bitter-tasting foods, it isn't the only reason. Sometimes children may not like the smell of a certain food or how it looks, but how it feels is often a stumbling block at this age. It is not uncommon for young children to refuse foods that are wet or slimy in some way. As I have mentioned previously, my firstborn refused any food in a sauce as soon as he hit toddlerhood, eschewing wet food for the accompanying dry breadsticks, crackers and toast at all opportunities. To this day, only one out of four of my children will eat mushrooms, not because of their taste, but their texture. Apparently, they are 'all squidgy' and make their teeth feel funny. I initially thought this was a strange quirk of my family until I realised how many others – not just children, but adults too – share this disdain.

Research into the eating habits of toddlers and preschoolers has found that the texture of food influences picky eating significantly more than colour or taste.[8] Further research has found a strong link between the sensory processing characteristics of children and the food that they eat, or rather don't eat.[9] For those children who do not have a specific sensory processing disorder (a specific condition where they struggle with sensory input), I wonder if this shunning of wet, slimy and squelchy foods in favour of their 'safe', dry counterparts is because of the way we speak about different textures as adults. Words like slimy and squelchy are used to describe monsters and aliens and other unpleasant creatures. Many parents can unconsciously pass on a fear of dirt to their children by constantly wiping their faces, or hands, whether it is to clean them of snot, ketchup, chocolate or mud. So our dislike of certain textures and the dirt and negativity associated with them must surely rub off on our children. Is this, perhaps, why so many of them avoid similar textures when it comes to eating?

Evolutionary eating

Many years ago, when we lived a hunter-gatherer lifestyle, or even a scavenger one, our eating would have been very different from how it is today, not just in terms of the actual food eaten, but also in the way we ate it. Our ancestors would not have had three regular meals a day, for their eating depended solely upon what they hunted, gathered or scavenged. Simply, they would have eaten when they could – when food was available. There would have been times of scant food offerings, when they would have gone several hours, if not days, without eating, followed by times of plenty, when they could eat to their hearts' content. And so it makes sense, when food is available, to eat as much as possible – a feast to counteract the famine that may be just around the corner. This opportunistic eating and intermittent fasting is in line with 5:2 eating – a trendy new healthy-eating ethos; however, toddlers and preschoolers have been doing it for years, long before anybody had even heard of 5:2. Quite simply, toddlers and preschoolers eat in the same way as our ancestors: feasting when they come across a food that they enjoy and fasting when there is nothing on offer that takes their fancy.

As a toddler, my daughter used to feast and fast every day, not dependent on the food on offer, but rather the time of day. She used to eat with gusto in the mornings – so much so that she would be on her third breakfast of the day by 10 a.m. and begging for lunch at eleven. But when the clock struck one, no more food would pass her lips until the next morning. At first, I panicked that she didn't eat anything in the afternoon and regularly turned her nose up at dinner. However, when I considered what she had eaten in the day, it was the same in terms of quantity as it would have been had she eaten at more 'regular' times. It just so happened that she did all her eating in a five-hour period, preferring to fast in the afternoons and evenings, ready for her next feast the following morning. We need to think about why we feel that our children must eat at certain times. Isn't the fact that they are eating what they need – whenever they eat it – more important?

Parental anxiety

As a parent of a previously picky eater, I understand how stressful it is. When my son was younger I spent hours every day worrying about his eating. I swung from thinking that he was somehow trying to manipulate me and was refusing to eat on purpose, to berating myself for being an awful parent. There were many times that I blamed myself. I felt that I had surely done something wrong. Had I made a mistake when weaning him? Was my cooking unpalatable? Was I placing too much pressure on him to eat? Or perhaps I needed to get stricter and force him to eat? I remember distinctly how hopeless it made me feel. Why couldn't I get him to eat? Would he ever eat again? Would he grow sick because of malnutrition? Would I be seen as a negligent parent? I bribed my son, begged him, scolded him when he didn't eat and spent hours cooking things to tempt him. If I had read or heard about a method somewhere, then I tried it. Nothing worked. With each failed attempt and discarded meal, I became more and more anxious, stressed and scared.

Ironically, I realise now that in stressing about my son's eating, I had created a self-fulfilling prophecy and made his eating even more picky. Research has shown that when mothers are concerned about their children undereating, they are more likely to pressure or bribe their children to eat[10] – behaviour which, in turn, is associated with an increase in picky eating. The more controlling I was around my son's eating, the less he ate. When I relaxed and just accepted him as he was, picky eating and all, I noticed a very small, positive effect on his eating. Lifting the pressure slowly encouraged him to eat a little more and, month by month, his pickiness began to subside. It was not a quick change by any means – it took several years until I no longer considered him 'picky' – but we were both happier and he did, eventually, grow out of it.

Solutions for picky eating

While being picky is completely normal and natural for young children, there are still several things that parents can do to slowly encourage less fussy eating. None of these is a 'quick-fix' solution; in fact, trying to rush any changes will ultimately backfire, making eating worse. So it is important that you have realistic expectations when it comes to a timeframe. Don't think in terms of days or even weeks, but months and years – although the results you do get, while slow to appear, will be the healthiest and most long-lasting. Remember, the goal of gentle eating is to create healthy eating habits for life.

Hold the praise and rewards

Praising a child for eating can be incredibly counterproductive. While the child may initially try to eat the food on offer, in order to earn lots of praise from their parents, the effect is unlikely to be long-lasting. And more worrying is how it encourages children to override their innate satiety cues in favour of pleasing their parent. Research has shown that children who are regularly praised for eating are statistically more likely to grow to be overweight in later life.[11] Being praised for eating encourages the child to associate it with feeling good. It is no surprise, then, that this emotional eating leads to disordered eating as the child grows and seeks to eat to make themselves feel better.

In a similar vein, rewarding for 'good eating' is also best avoided. Rewards may temporarily make a child eat more, but they can also have a negative effect on whether the child actually likes the food and can cause an aversion to previously liked foods.[12] This unintended negative outcome is even more likely to occur if the reward on offer is another food, for instance if the child is rewarded with ice cream for eating their broccoli.

Eating really should be emotion-free. That means no praise and no rewards. The goal of gentle eating is to raise a child who has a healthy relationship with food, one who eats when they are hungry and stops when they are full and considers all food as fuel, not 'naughty' or 'good'. When we reward or praise a child for 'eating up', clearing their plate or even trying something, we encourage them to override their own bodily cues. They may temporarily eat a little more, or try something green, but this does not mean you are instilling good eating habits. As a parent, your role is to stay neutral about the food the child eats. That means you don't reward or praise when they eat 'well' and you don't admonish them if they don't eat something either.

Remove the pressure

When your child doesn't eat, or constantly refuses a certain food, it can be really hard to not prompt them to 'just try one forkful' or comment negatively that they 'never try anything'. Gentle eating is about taking a responsive, compassionate and authoritative approach – that means taking a step back and allowing the child to take more control over their eating. It can be easy to slip into an authoritarian style of parenting when you are worried about your child's eating, but the pressure that comes with such an approach will always mean it backfires. Research has shown that children who are pressured to eat by their parents eat significantly less than those who are not, and they are more likely to avoid the foods that they are being pressured to eat.[13] So while you may be tempted to cajole your child into taking just one more bite, the best way to reduce picky eating is to keep quiet and remove any pressure. If you feel the need to say something, then saying, 'You don't have to eat it if you don't want to' is far more empowering and far more likely to result in a positive outcome.

Don't give up

As children grow, their tastes change, and their dislike of bitter foods, in particular, will subside a little. Liking a food is not only related to taste though. A child's experiences will also affect which foods they choose to eat. For this reason, one of the most powerful things you can do is to keep re-presenting the challenging food. There is a myth that it takes ten or fifteen exposures to a food for a child to try it or begin to like it. Aside from the fact that it's mentioned in thousands of articles, books and websites (unattributed to any source), I can find no evidence for this. In reality, it may take hundreds of exposures before your child attempts and, ultimately, likes a certain food. It may take years. How often have you heard an adult say things like, 'I hated Brussels sprouts as a child. I didn't start eating them until I was in my twenties'? Research does show that repeated exposure to a food increases the chance that a child will eat it, but it is important that you remember to stay calm and avoid placing any pressure on them to actually try it.[14] I find the best way to approach repeated food exposure is to accept that it will almost always result in repeated refusal. And if you don't expect your child to try the food, then you are not disappointed when they don't, which, in turn, helps to keep your stress levels down. If they do try it, then it is a happy miracle!

One step at a time

When it comes to types of food that you know your child isn't keen on, offering only one of them at a time provides the least stress for you and your child. So if your child usually refuses green vegetables, for example, only serve one type. Putting cabbage and peas on their plate at the same time is likely to lead to anxiety and stress for you both. Presenting just peas, or just cabbage, however, is likely to be much more successful. In addition to only offering one challenging food at a time, make sure you always offer something that you know your child *will* eat. Their plate should ideally always comprise one new or challenging food, one that they are neutral about and one that they are almost guaranteed to eat. Being presented with food in this manner means the child should feel more relaxed – and a more relaxed child is one who is more likely to try something new or challenging. Remember to remain emotionless about what your child chooses to eat. Don't prompt them to try the new food or praise them for eating the challenging food.

Give them some control

Gentle eating is about empowering your children and respecting their likes and dislikes, satiety and hunger. In essence, this means giving them control over their eating. As adults, we may not realise how little control our children have over their food intake on a daily basis, because we take the control over our own eating for granted. Giving your child more say over their eating can be a wonderfully empowering way to reduce pickiness and increase food intake. Most importantly, you need to honour your child's likes and dislikes. Too often, parents unconsciously try to force their own food preferences onto their children. Comments such as 'Don't be silly, it's lovely' can quickly creep into your daily dialogue without you realising. It's OK for children to like foods that we don't and dislike foods that we may love.

A lovely way to honour your child's dislikes and give them more control is to place an empty bowl on the table when you eat. Call it the 'unwanted food bowl', and if anybody in your family really doesn't like something on their plate and doesn't want to try it, they are allowed to put it in the unwanted food bowl, no questions asked. Similarly, using serving bowls that children can serve themselves from, rather than you putting food directly on their plates, allows them to select the food they would like in differing amounts.

As well as likes and dislikes, we must honour our children's hunger and satiety. If we want to raise children with healthy eating habits, we must understand how important it is for them to recognise and respect their bodies' cues. If a child only eats a few mouthfuls and then declares that they're not hungry, far too often we reply with something like: 'Of course, you're hungry. You haven't eaten for ages and you've been running around all afternoon. You need to eat, so eat up.' We deny them the opportunity to self-regulate their eating. Around 85 per cent of parents prompt their children to eat regularly, an alarming figure considering that children whose parents overly control their food intake in early childhood grow to favour high-fat and high-energy foods, struggle to control their eating and have a more restrictive diet than those who were given the freedom to eat in line with their own preferences and satiation levels.[15]

Allowing your child to control their own eating – both what they eat and how much of it – may seem like a scary concept and many parents worry that their child will accidentally starve, or consume only food with low nutrient levels, but scientists have found that young children actually eat a fairly well-balanced diet when left to their own devices.[16] Although food intake at individual mealtimes may be erratic, young children do seem to eat a well-balanced diet when their food consumption over a twenty-four-hour period is calculated.

Time to get messy!

For children who struggle with the sensory aspects of eating, especially foods that are slimy, mushy and gooey, incorporating more messy play into their days, focusing on the sensations that they struggle with, can help them with food acceptance.

Research has shown that sensory play with real fruits and vegetables can have a positive impact on children's fruit and vegetable consumption.[17] The experiment, conducted with three- and four-year-olds, found that children who had played with fruit and vegetables in a messy play session tried significantly more of them than those who had not. This finding proved true not only for the specific fruit and vegetables that they had played with, but also those that they hadn't.

Parents of children who struggle with getting messy, and often avoid 'messy foods' as a result, should also focus on their own behaviour. If you are overly clean, you can unconsciously pass on a fear of 'mess' to your children. Parents who make a dash for the baby wipes as soon as their toddler puts their hands in their food, or when they get as much of what they are eating on their face as in their mouth, can cause their child to become anxious about making a mess with food. In turn, this may lead to picky eating, especially when it comes to food with messier textures. If you can identify yourself in this, try to find a way to keep the baby wipes in the packet and postpone the hand-washing. When you do clean up your child, be careful to not use words like 'messy' or 'mucky', instead saying something like, 'Wow, you look like you enjoyed that! You were so excited to eat it; it's gone everywhere!'

Picture perfect

Imagine that you are on holiday and are served something that you don't recognise. You don't speak the language, so are unable to ascertain what the food is; all you know is that it doesn't look like anything you have ever seen or eaten before. Would you be just a little reluctant to try it? Now imagine living this scenario every day and I think you'll begin to understand how toddlers and preschoolers feel.

Helping children to familiarise themselves with new and different foods can help to reduce neophobia and any anxiety surrounding them. Research has found that looking at books containing pictures of food helps toddlers to be more adventurous when trying them for the first time.[18] Together with a parent, children aged between nineteen and twenty-six months looked at a book containing pictures of unfamiliar fruits or vegetables every day for two weeks. At the end of the fortnight, researchers determined whether the book exposure had had any impact on the eating behaviour of the children. They found that it had, significantly so, with the toddlers consuming more of the unfamiliar vegetables they had seen in the book, when compared to others that they had not seen. This research has wonderful implications for parents. If you can find a book with one of your child's favourite characters as well, I suspect the result would be even more powerful.

Mirror, mirror

Children learn how to behave by mimicking us. They watch us day in, day out and look to us to learn what to do in different situations, eating being one of them.

As a parent, your eating behaviours and likes and dislikes are paramount when it comes to influencing your child's preferences. Think about the message you are giving to your child when you take the crusts off your bread, push your vegetables around your plate or ask a restaurant to 'hold the salad'. Think too about what you convey when you refer to sweet foods as 'yummy', 'naughty' or 'a treat'.

Research has shown that toddlers and preschoolers are more likely to try a new food if an adult is eating the same food at the same time.[19] Further research has found that this –'modelling' – is the most successful way of encouraging a child to eat.[20] Modelling has a more significant impact on child eating than prompting them to eat, rewarding them or rationalising with them about eating ('You need to eat your vegetables to be healthy; if you don't eat them, you won't grow big and strong.').

The problem with modelling is that as well as eating the same food at the same time, it also requires us, as parents, to slow down and sit down to eat with our children, something that often doesn't happen if parents work and the children are at day care. Try to find time to eat at least one meal every day with your child and at weekends aim for all meals. If you are not eating your meal at the same time as your child, serve yourself a small snack of the foods that your child is struggling with and eat that with them. Modelling really does have such a powerful effect on toddler and preschooler eating that it is worth making the time to do it as often as possible.

Honour their inner caveman

Earlier in this chapter we discussed the opportunistic eating and intermittent fasting patterns commonly followed by young children (see page 111). While this eating pattern is entirely normal and quite healthy, it is clearly at odds with the modern construct of 'three square meals a day'. If you have a toddler or a preschooler who suits the eating patterns of the Paleolithic era far more than those of the twenty-first century, the easiest solution is to swap your modern eating expectations for something more instinctive and in keeping with their habits. Allowing your child to eat at any time they feel hunger usually results in them eating significantly more and usually more healthily than if you try to make them fit in with socially accepted mealtimes. And one of the best ways to accomplish this is to embrace the idea of a grazing tray.

Grazing trays are simply containers of some description containing a variety of foods that the child can select from whenever they feel the need to eat. They may return to the tray frequently and eat little and often throughout the course of the day, in a 'gatherer' style, or they may eat a large quantity far less frequently, mimicking more of a 'hunter' style. Either way, the amount consumed over a twenty-four-hour period is usually more than they would have eaten at regular breakfast, lunch and dinner times, especially if you also mirror eating the same foods.

To make a grazing tray you need an appropriate container – one with individual compartments tends to work best, or you can buy special plates with different compartments. The insert from a fishing or tool box works very well too and is usually much cheaper, or a couple of large ice-cube trays also work. The aim is to fill each compartment with a different food. Suggestions for foods that work well are:

- carrot sticks

- cucumber batons

- cherry tomatoes cut in half

- sweet pepper strips

- grapes cut in half

- raisins

- mini breadsticks and hummus

- cubes of cheese

- hard-boiled eggs, quartered

- mini falafels

- sushi rolls (without raw fish)

- ham or chicken strips

- fresh, raw peas

- mini crackers with cheese spread

- strawberries, blueberries, raspberries and blackberries

- apple and pear slices

- edamame beans

- pickles

- mini sandwiches

- avocado strips

- cold penne pasta tubes

- sweetcorn kernels

- cashew nuts and walnuts.

At the start of each day, place freshly prepared food in the tray and leave it where your child has free and easy access. Independent access is an important feature of the grazing tray, which usually rules out storing it in the fridge. (Most toddlers and preschoolers are unable to easily open a fridge door and take a tray out without adult assistance.) As the tray will not be chilled, be sure not to put it near a radiator or fire. It will usually be fine to leave most foods out for three or four hours without them spoiling, but you may well need to refresh the contents two or three times each day. You may also consider resting the tray on cool packs to prolong the life of the food.

When you first begin to use a grazing tray, it may not seem as if your child is eating very much. However, if you keep track of what you have put out each day, you will probably find that they have eaten significantly more than you thought. Some parents use a grazing tray in place of all meals; others use them just for the middle of the day, offering a regular breakfast in the morning and dinner at the end of the day. Whichever way you use them, grazing trays are an effective, child-friendly and gentle way to encourage healthier eating.

Full focus

All too often, our busy lives mean that we eat on the run. We rarely focus fully on eating, and yet this is exactly what is needed if we want to encourage good habits in our children. Eating with full focus means being more aware of our body's hunger and satiety cues. It encourages mindful eating, whereas distracted eating encourages the opposite.

Whether they are sitting at a table to eat a full meal or grazing from a selection of foods throughout the day, children should eat with their full focus on their food: that means no snacks in a buggy, lunch on the go in the car, or eating in front of the television or while being entertained by other screens or toys. It also means that food is not used to distract them from potentially difficult behaviour. The big emotions underlying the difficult behaviour mean that children will never be able to fully concentrate on eating, while the use of food as a distraction technique is not only poor discipline but potentially encourages disordered, emotional eating in the future.

Knowing that children mirror our eating behaviour, parents should be especially aware of where their own focus is during eating. This means turning off the television, shutting the laptop and putting down your mobile phone to focus fully on your own food.

Try to relax

Being the mother of a non-eater or a fussy eater is certainly the most difficult aspect of parenting I had to face. No other issue has affected me quite so much or made me feel so utterly hopeless. And with that hopelessness came self-doubt, guilt and heaps of anxiety.

Anxiety is catching. No matter how much I tried to approach mealtimes with a smile on my face, my son could sense my dread. Of course, he picked up on it, my anxiety feeding his own eating anxiety in a never-ending cycle. Research has confirmed that parental anxiety is associated with fussy eating in preschoolers.[21] And the same is undoubtedly true for toddlers. Worrying about your child not eating makes you anxious which, in turn, creates a self-fulfilling prophecy whereby the child does not eat. It is a cycle that must be broken.

As I mentioned earlier (see page 118), my son's eating ultimately improved when I managed to relax and go with it. I accepted my son for all he was, picky eating and all. In so doing, I took the pressure off him and off myself. I dropped my expectations to a level where I was pleased if he ate anything, even one tiny nibble or crumb. I ditched the praise, the rewards, the pressure, the prompting and I just let him be. I made eating unemotional. I took deep breaths before every meal and reminded myself it was OK if he didn't eat it. It wasn't about me – I was not failing. I was doing the best I could. I won't pretend it was easy. It wasn't. But the more I practised my new-found Zen-like demeanour, the easier it was to step into those chilled-out shoes for real – until, ultimately, I found I wasn't pretending any more. The calmer I became, the more my son ate. It wasn't quick, but there was change and I was happy with any tiny speck of hope.

Other common toddler and preschooler eating concerns

While picky eating is the most universal issue with toddler and preschooler eating, it is by no means the only worry of parents of one- to four-year-olds. There are a few other concerns that are raised quite frequently, namely worries about table manners (or rather, lack of them), how to cope when your child wants to eat all the time, what to do when pudding holds far more interest than savoury food and what to do when children are in day care where eating is approached in a different way. Let's take a look at each of these in turn.

Table manners

Young children and table manners are not necessarily terms you would commonly associate with each other. Despite this, table manners remain a top concern among parents the world over, whether it's about children throwing food, playing with food, not using cutlery, refusing to sit in a high chair, making strange noises while eating or refusing to sit still while others finish eating.

Before we look at how to cope with specific issues surrounding table manners, we must consider whether or not our expectations of young children are appropriate for their age. As adults, we can understand social rules and niceties, we appreciate the consequences of not following them and we can empathise with others who may be offended by non-compliance. We also have the neurological development necessary to control our own impulses and behaviour, meaning that we can stop ourselves from doing something if we feel that others may perceive our actions as rude. Toddlers and preschoolers are not like us. Their brains are still developing and the last part of the brain to develop is the area responsible for impulse control and emotional intelligence. The intricate social expectations that underpin table manners will not truly be understood until this has occurred, between the ages of eleven and twenty-one. We must stop expecting young children to think and behave like us; until we do, we are going to be continually disappointed and stressed by their behaviour. Table manners are an advanced skill beyond what most toddlers and preschoolers can understand and manage.

Does this mean that there is nothing that you can do? Do you have to live with your mini caveman and their uncouth eating for the next ten to twenty years? Not quite. Modelling remains the most powerful way to teach children. If you make your expectations clear and consistently model the behaviour you want to see, then there is a high chance that your child will mirror you. This doesn't mean that they have the same grasp of table manners as you, but it does mean that you can curb their caveman tendencies superficially, until they are old enough to understand the intricacies themselves.

How to get your child to use cutlery

Cutlery is quite a strange invention. If you think of all the other primates in the world, they all eat with their 'hands'. Indeed, humans ate food with their hands for centuries. Hands are perfectly designed for eating. Our opposable thumbs and pincer grips mean that we can pick up anything and eat it with ease. From an evolutionary perspective, we have no need for knives, forks and spoons. Toddlers and preschoolers are often far more adept at eating with their hands than with cutlery, which can often slow down their eating and cause frustration. It is not surprising, therefore, that many choose to ditch it and dive in with their hands instead.

If you do want to encourage your child to use cutlery sooner rather than later, then there are two important points to consider. First, you must choose cutlery that is easy for them to use. Most adult silverware is not appropriate for a young child; similarly, many items designed for young children are also not optimal. When choosing cutlery for a toddler or preschooler, you must consider the sizing – not too small or too large. The ideal size (including the handle) is around one and a half times the length of their hand. You also need to think about the circumference of the handles. Choosing cutlery with chunkier handles enables a better grip and makes manoeuvring easier. Also, think about starting out with simplified cutlery. For instance, you can buy a 'spork', a cross between a spoon and a fork, which allows the child to do more, while only having to focus on manipulating one piece of cutlery. The second point to consider is, once again, mirroring. If you want your child to use cutlery at all times, then you have to do so yourself. Do you sometimes eat chips with a fork, but at other times out of a bag, with your fingers? This inconsistency is confusing for children. You must always demonstrate the behaviour you want your child to display.

How to get your child to stop throwing food

If you have a child who throws, rather than eats, their food, you may despair over what you have done to raise such a little hooligan. And you wouldn't be alone in your despair. Throwing food is universal. All children do it at some point. Some may only throw food once, some may throw it every day, but they all do it. It's important to understand why.

The most obvious answer is because they don't want to eat it. Giving a child food when they are not hungry is significantly more likely to result in the food being thrown; similarly, giving a child too much food often has the same result. Here, the answer is to be mindful of your child's hunger and satiety levels and to respect their appetite. Don't put more food on their plate than they will realistically eat, and if they tell you that they are full, respect that and remove the food. Throwing also occurs when the child doesn't like the food they have been given. Previously, I have mentioned placing a bowl on the table in which they can put food that they don't want on their plate (see page 123). If you don't give them an alternative, then the only solution, as far as they are concerned, is to throw unwanted food. Throwing food also gets your attention if you are preoccupied and your child is trying to signal to you that they are done or not ready to eat. Focusing more on your child at mealtimes should hopefully avoid this.

We must also consider that throwing is fun, at least for the child. Throwing food could be an indication that your child needs more active play. Recognising this and saying, 'You want to throw! You can't throw your food, but let's go into the garden and throw a ball,' is much more effective than simply telling the child to stop throwing.

Finally, throwing is a normal developmental stage in toddlerhood and the preschool years. As we learned in the previous chapter, children learn and develop skills by practising them, a process known as schemas (see page 88). There are several different schemas that children must experience in order to learn, each related to a different skill and activity. The trajectory schema is responsible for teaching children about the properties of objects when they are thrown and how gravity works. While it is frustrating for parents to clean up after constant food throwing, for the child it is a wonderful learning opportunity, akin to a laboratory experiment. Of course, throwing food is not acceptable, but you should recognise that your child needs to do it. Once again, offering to take them outside to throw a ball instead, or throwing soft beanbags inside, can help to fulfil this need.

What to do when your child won't sit in their high chair

If you have been using a high chair for your child since they were a baby, they will probably, at some point, refuse to sit in it. While high chairs may be more convenient for parents, they don't provide a good modelling opportunity for children. If your child sees you sitting on a regular chair at the table, they are likely to want to copy you. Similarly, if you eat your sandwich while sitting on the sofa, it is understandable that your child will be upset when you try to sit them in their high chair to eat theirs. And toddlers, food and sofas are a bad mix, for obvious reasons!

One great way that I have found to overcome high-chair refusal is to eat with your children on a large mat or plastic tablecloth or oilcloth on the floor – something I call carpet picnics. My children have always loved doing this. When they were small, picnics were always guaranteed to hold their attention and they would eat more than they may have done otherwise. (When I say more, I don't mean overeating – rather, picnics reduced picky eating.) Carpet picnics turned a potentially stressful scenario into one that was altogether happier and more relaxed.

How to get your child to stop making strange noises at mealtimes

Some toddlers and preschoolers can make a lot of noise while eating. Sometimes this is simply because they eat with their mouths open; at other times the noises are made deliberately and often involve grunting, lip smacking and even growling. The best way to encourage children to keep their mouths closed when they are eating is to model this yourself and tell them what you want them to do, very clearly – not what you *don't* want them to do. It is far better to say to your child, 'Can you close your mouth so that your lips touch each other when you eat?' rather than, 'Stop eating with your mouth open'.

Deliberate noises often stem from anxiety and attention seeking. If a child is uncomfortable with the food, but feels there is no other way to attract your attention – especially if you are busy talking to your partner or another child – they quickly discover ways in which to do so. The simple answer is to focus more on your child while they are eating and reduce any possible distractions at mealtimes.

Sometimes strange noises are just the child's show of appreciation. Whereas you and I may say, 'Hmm, this food is lovely!' toddlers and preschoolers may hum, growl and loudly smack their lips. While the noise itself may be irritating and slightly odd, it is well meant and even a compliment. Try to focus more on their enjoyment and not the noise. Say, 'You like the food! It's yummy isn't it?' This helps the child to find the words to voice their appreciation, which, ultimately, will make the noises redundant.

What to do when your child won't remain at the table while others are eating

As adults, we understand that it is rude to leave the table when others are eating. As boring as it may be to continue sitting 'nicely' when we have finished eating, we know that it is inappropriate to leave the table and, with our adult brains, we are able to overcome our impulses to get up and go. Expecting one- to four-year-olds to mimic this behaviour, however, is pretty unrealistic. Toddlers and preschoolers don't think like us and they cannot control their impulses. We may consider it rude when they leave the table while we are still eating, but they don't. This is one problem for which, unfortunately, there is no solution – at least not when it comes to changing the child. Really, it is the adult who has the problem here, and the easiest solution is to readjust expectations accordingly. The only way to keep a child at the table after they have finished eating is to entertain them in some way – colouring or perhaps playing on a phone or tablet. Neither of these encourage good habits around eating, as they both take the focus away from hunger and satiety and potentially create far worse problems than they solve. The best answer is to accept that toddlers and preschoolers aren't adults and allow them to leave the table when they have finished. As they grow and their brains develop they will understand why it is rude to leave the table when others haven't finished and they will have the impulse control necessary to remain there. In the meantime, they will learn from you by observing your behaviour. You are already teaching them by remaining at the table yourself. In time, they will copy you.

What to do when your child plays with their food

While playing with food is seen as the height of rudeness in adults, it is actually a sign of good learning in toddlers and preschoolers. Children learn about food and eating via all of their senses, taste being only one of them. It is important that children take in all of the sensory stimulation food provides – that means smell, sight and, importantly, touch, as well as taste. Research has found that when children play with their food and get messy, it increases their learning.[22] Scientists have found that toddlers are able to learn the names of the food that they are exposed to more easily and quickly when they are allowed to play with it, and we know that familiarity with food means children are more likely to eat it.

The child who never stops eating

As mentioned earlier, by far the most common worry surrounding eating in the toddler and preschooler years is picky eating. For some families, however, their concern couldn't be more different – they are worried that their child eats too much.

When my second son was a baby, he had what I would call a 'big appetite'. He would eat anything he was offered and people frequently commented on how much food he consumed. As my firstborn was similar as a baby, but quickly turned into 'the boy who wouldn't eat' as a toddler, I was expecting the same with my second son. Only it never happened. He continued to eat 'like a horse'. He was the opposite of fussy. I never found a food he wouldn't eat. He always seemed to be hungry. If we went out for the day, I had to prepare by packing a bag full of snacks for him. At first, I was happy. I felt relaxed and content to be blessed with a 'good eater' after the stress of my non-eating firstborn. That happiness soon began to give way to anxiety, however. Did he eat too much? Had I somehow created an eating problem that would see him binge his way through life? Was he going to be obese? Would he be sick from eating so much? He was always slightly big for his age, although that was reflected in his height as well as his weight. I pushed my worries aside and tried to convince myself that he knew his body better than I did. I tried my hardest to trust him and allow him to eat when he decided he was hungry. By the time he started school his eating had started to slow a little, as had his growth. He was incredibly active and quickly turned into a healthy, lithe, sporty little boy with no weight problems. To this day, he has a good relationship with food and, if anything, as a teenager, he is slightly on the skinny side. My anxiety about his constant eating was unfounded, and I remain happy with my decision to allow him to control his own food intake and trust in him knowing what his body needed.

I sometimes think we are scared when we have children who eat a lot, especially in the early years, as picky eating is so common. Ironically, we may believe that children who *do* eat have a problem when compared to their pickier peers. But the reality is that both are entirely normal. If children are otherwise healthy and not significantly overweight, with plenty of opportunities to move their bodies, then it is always better to trust that they know their own needs better than we do.

When dessert is more appealing than dinner

In Chapter 2, I we looked at the disordered eating habits of many adults, one of which is our labelling of food as 'good' and 'naughty' and giving sweet foods personalities. As adults, we view dessert as an unnecessary but palatable add-on to our main meal. Dessert is a treat and something that is put on a pedestal – a reward for eating our more boring and less appealing savoury food. Too often, parents tell their children that they can't have their dessert until they have eaten up their main meal. When children are denied dessert until they have cleaned their plate, it encourages them to overeat and override their satiety levels. Simply, they continue to eat their meal when they are not hungry in order to get dessert. The very idea of dessert encourages mindless eating.

What if dessert was not treated as special? What if it was treated as just food – not something that happens as 'a little treat' after the 'healthy' food is eaten? Would it still hold such power over us? I don't think so. And what would happen if your child was allowed to eat their dessert before or at the same time as their main meal? It may seem a bizarre idea, but no more bizarre than the social diktat of always eating sweet things after a meal. If you truly trust your child to eat when they are hungry and stop when they are full, a small and non-filling dessert is not going to stop them eating the rest of their food; but it might just stop them from wolfing down food that they are not really hungry for in order to get the reward of dessert afterwards. It could also help to release the hold that sweet foods have over so many of us.

Eating at day care and preschool

While gentle-eating principles arguably produce the healthiest relationships with food, there is no getting away from the fact that they are not part of a mainstream approach. It is ironic that something that is the closest to guaranteeing an emotionally and physically healthy individual is still a fringe, or alternative, movement. One of the areas in which this is really brought home is in day-care and education settings. In the next chapter, we will look at the impact of schools upon childhood eating, but for now we should look at how to marry gentle eating and day care.

The first and most important thing I can say to you regarding your child's day care is that it is a service you are paying for and, as such, you are perfectly entitled to question it. We wouldn't accept having to compromise our ideals when buying a car or a house, so why do we accept it when it comes to how our children are cared for in our absence? When we are expecting a baby, we spend time writing a birth plan, listing our wishes and beliefs, so that they can be followed by professionals when we give birth. Why then don't we continue this trend to communicate with any caregivers once our children are born? Remembering that gentle eating is not mainstream, the chances are that you will need to spend some time explaining your choices and beliefs to your child's caregiver, backing those beliefs with evidence (the studies that you will find listed in the References are a good starting point – see page 213). It is likely that your childcare setting already has an established feeding schedule, but never be afraid to ask if they could follow your child's individual needs. The following are some examples of things you may wish to include in your childcare plan, concerning eating:

- Please don't prompt my child to eat something or praise him when he has done so.

- Please don't encourage my child to eat more than he chooses to. It is important to us that he is allowed to stop eating when he senses that he is full.

- If my child asks for food and you don't believe that he is hungry, please try to trust his hunger cues and respond to them.

- Please do not reward or praise my child for eating all his food, clearing his plate or eating something he doesn't normally eat.

- If my child indicates that he is not hungry at a normal meal-time, please respect that he knows his body's hunger and satiety cues and don't encourage him to eat.

- Please consider letting my child snack outside of regular meal-time if he indicates that he is hungry.

- Please don't withhold pudding until my child has eaten all of his main meal. We don't want to encourage him to eat more than he needs in order to receive the reward of something sweet.

- Please do offer my child foods that he usually refuses, but please do not make a big deal of it if he doesn't touch them.

- Please do not point out other children who have 'eaten well' to my child; modelling is powerful and it may encourage him to overeat to receive praise.

Perhaps the most important thing to highlight to any child-care provider is that you do not hold them responsible if your child doesn't eat very much. The role of a nursery worker, child-minder or nanny is to keep the child happy and healthy and safe in their care and, just like parents, many can worry that they have not done their best for the child if they haven't eaten much. Concern about picky eating and undereating is common among day-care workers, just as it is for parents. Your role is also to reassure and reaffirm here. Perhaps lending this book once you are finished with it would be a good start.

Questions from parents

I'm going to close this chapter with some questions sent to me by parents of toddlers and preschoolers, struggling with certain elements of their child's eating. I hope that these, together with my answers, will help to bring some of the issues discussed in this chapter to life.

Q. *We have seventeen-month-old twin boys. We started them on food from around six months, initially in the form of home-made purées and then some finger foods. One twin has transitioned well to eating solids of all types. The other steadfastly refuses and will still only eat purées, mainly of fruit and yoghurt. He will sometimes eat veggie purées if they are relatively sweet – like carrot, sweet potato or butternut squash – but not always. He won't ever accept meat or fish. He is highly tactile with solid food and will feel it and turn it over in his hands for a while, but almost always reject it again* *(he often appears to strongly dislike the 'feel' of something). We are tackling this by exposing him at every mealtime to different foods, solids and purées, and letting him explore different things, never forcing him to eat, and we always try to eat evening meals together as a family. We've been doing all of this for many months now with no change and are not sure what else we can try other than continuing as we are and giving him time. He is growing, but he's small for his age and doesn't seem to be catching up.*

Any advice or other ideas on things we can try would be much appreciated.

A. It sounds as if you are doing a great job already by not forcing your son to eat and modelling the eating you would like to see from him by eating as a family. You *will* see results from this, but it may take a lot longer than you would expect or hope for. Real change could take years, rather than weeks or months. There are a few things that I will suggest you try, which may help to speed up some change but, even then, it is important that you stay focused on the longer, rather than shorter term.

First, I would recommend that you work a little to help your son to get the sensory input from food that he obviously needs. We know that toddlers are more likely to eat a food if they have been exposed to it in a safe and unpressured way before they are expected to eat it. The best way to do this is via play and reading. I'd suggest setting up sensory play sessions with some foods, particularly fruit and vegetables, well away from mealtimes. If there are any particular foods that your son struggles with, including them would be a good idea. For instance, you could grate some cauliflower to create 'rice' that he can get his fingers into, making sure that you grate it in front of him so he sees it in its original form first. You might try printing with paint and slices of courgette, pepper, cucumber and apple. Or you could create a scene with some model dinosaurs or other animals, containing broccoli trees, grass made from squashed peas and mountains from cubes of potatoes. It's important that he can really get stuck in to touching different foods, not just in play but when he's actually eating too. In fact, what we consider 'playing with food' at mealtimes is an important learning opportunity for children, so don't discourage his sensory exploration at mealtimes. I'd also recommend that you find some picture books featuring different fruit and vegetables and help to familiarise your son with the foods in the book before presenting them to him at mealtimes.

We know that repeated exposure to foods is a key factor in acceptance, but it may take more attempts than you think – hundreds rather than tens. Always aim to include an item of food that has been previously rejected and perhaps one that is new at each meal, but also include a 'safe' food that you know your son will eat. This safe food helps to take the pressure off him, as he knows that there is something he can eat. If he gets distressed about something you have given him, reassure him that he doesn't have to eat it if he doesn't want to and give him the option to take it off his plate if he prefers.

I can imagine it is stressful for you to have one twin who is a 'good eater' and one who isn't, but do try to never compare the two and, importantly, never praise his brother for eating well. You need to keep your feelings about your boys' eating neutral. On this note, your feelings really matter. The more anxious you become about your son's eating, the more likely it is that the pattern will continue. Finding a way to allay and calm your nerves is critical. Your sons – both of them – are eating normally for their age and it sounds like you're doing a great job parenting them. I think it's time to give yourself a break. I understand your son is small for his age, but somebody must be. The law of averages means, by definition, that some children are bigger than average and others are smaller. That's OK. It doesn't matter if he's on the second, fiftieth or ninety-ninth centile and he doesn't have to be on the same centile as his brother. Sometimes accepting that you have a 'little eater' is far more powerful than trying to change them.

Q. *My two-year-old daughter will very rarely stay seated at the table to eat her meal. She is full of energy all the time and since ditching the high chair and booster seat I can't keep her at the table. To be honest, even when she was restrained by the high chair, she'd be constantly escaping the straps and standing up trying to get out, so I guess she's never liked being constrained. Her cot was rejected for similar reasons, but that's another story!*

At home I let her get up and down and eat as and when she feels like it. I've become a lot more relaxed about her eating habits recently and now pretty much go with the flow. She eats well over the course of twenty-four hours, so I figure it's not worth the battle. Until, that is, we go to eat at someone else's house. Then I feel mortified! We were at a friend's last night and her two girls sat nicely at the table until they'd finished eating . . . my daughter ate some, got down, had a play, returned, and I could almost see the horror my friend was trying to mask at my letting her do this. Should I be trying to enforce better table manners? If so, how? She is very strong-willed and determined, so confining her without physical restraints is something of a challenge!

A. High chairs are a strange invention. I'm not keen on them either. Some children are happy in them and if they are, then that's great. But for those children who dislike them, I think trying to insist on them using one is fighting a losing battle.

So I totally agree with the idea of ditching yours, but what I would try to change is your daughter's lack of attention when it comes to eating. At only two years old she is going to struggle to keep still for long, but by allowing her to play and eat on the move, you take away her focus on eating. This means that she may miss her satiety cues and overeat if she is busy playing. Obviously, this is not a great eating habit to encourage as she gets older – it's akin to us eating while playing on our phone. I would therefore try to enforce a boundary whereby it's OK that she doesn't sit in the high chair to eat, but that when she *does* eat she needs to sit down and focus on what she is doing. If she wants to play, then that's fine, but she doesn't play *and* eat.

Two things that I think would work well for you are the idea of carpet picnics and grazing trays. The idea with the former is that toys go away and the two of you sit on the mat and eat, focusing on your food, talking to each other about it and observing each other. If she gets up, then I would remind her that if she still wants to eat, she should sit down. If she wants to play, then that's OK too, but the food needs to go away, albeit temporarily until she says that she is hungry again. I would also recommend the idea of a grazing tray – a selection of food you have prepared, left out in a tray or plate with different compartments. This allows your daughter to snack throughout the day when she is hungry and then return to her previous, or a new, activity when she is full. My boundary would be the same here though: when she eats she needs to focus on eating, so I would encourage her to put down the toy she is playing with.

In terms of your friend's children, I do find that many – if not most – adults have unrealistic expectations of toddlers when it comes to table manners. I am not a fan of children sitting at the table until everybody has finished their food. I think it is a bizarre social ritual that toddlers just cannot grasp. There is also a chance that it could lead to overeating if children are made to sit at the table and eat for a specific period of time. I would have no issue with your daughter leaving the table when she is done, and really don't think it is anything you should worry about, whether you are at home or at a friend's house. As before, however, I would suggest that she doesn't yo-yo between play and eating at the table. I wonder if this was what your friend was more concerned about, especially given the powerful effect of modelling and the influence that your daughter may have had on her children? I guess you won't really know, but what I have learned in my years as a parent is that it is far better to focus on your own children and not worry about what others think of them!

Q. *My son is now two years and three months old. We began weaning him onto solids at five months, as he was starting to try to steal food off my plate. We began with spoon-feeding, as I hadn't heard of baby-led weaning at the time. He was a good eater from the get-go. I would make my own fruit and vegetable purées and freeze them in ice-cube trays. I began trying him with finger foods at seven months, but only with mixed success. He loved bread, crackers and cookies, and he was also fine with pieces of chicken, but anything involving vegetables or fruit he would poke at but very rarely put in his mouth. He also didn't display a lot of interest in putting his fingers in puréed food.*

By the time he was halfway proficient with his spoon, it became apparent that he was an unusually neat child. I don't know if some of this has transferred from me. I am a bit obsessive about food messes, so when we started weaning I would have a cloth handy and clean up as we went. But then I read that this was not a good idea, and that babies should just make whatever mess they want with food and it can be cleaned up after. So I did try hard to rein in my habits, but he just stayed tidy. Any food messes he made were always accidental/clumsy and there was and still is very little mess that he makes intentionally with food. He continues to have an aversion to touching puréed food, and while he doesn't freak out if some of it gets on him, he doesn't engage in that sort of behaviour voluntarily.

The sensory sensitivity extends beyond food. He has always been a cautious child. We had minimal problems with him putting inappropriate stuff in his mouth and he rarely tries to eat things that fall on the floor. He has never been a fan of messy play. If he gets his hands dirty in the playground, he immediately tries to wipe them.

I am not particularly worried. He does not become unduly agitated overall, and I can see that he's slowly overcoming some hesitation on his own over time. We don't force him to interact with or eat stuff he rejects. We don't operate a clean-plate policy, but we do try and encourage him to keep eating if he stops. If he is refusing emphatically, we reduce our demands on him – eat three more spoons or two more pieces, etc. Mostly, we do this not to make sure he eats everything, but as a way of keeping in place the boundaries around certain activities that he demands to do all the time (watching TV, for example) – i.e. that these things happen after dinner. So if he refuses to eat because he wants to watch TV, we always try to have a successful negotiation whereby he eats X amount more and then he can watch a little bit of TV. Sometimes he cooperates and sometimes he doesn't.

My questions are, is this normal, or did I make it worse somehow with our food habits? And will he grow out of this, or is there anything else you'd recommend other than continuing to introduce various forms of sensory play?

A. I think there are two separate aspects to consider here, the first being the sensory issues and the second being your eating boundaries.

Starting with the sensory issues, some children – and adults too – are simply not fans of mess or dirt and that's OK. It's when this reaches a point that it negatively impacts other areas of life that we should be concerned. It doesn't sound as if you are hugely anxious about your son's eating, but if you are concerned about his food intake, or pickiness or, alternatively, if you find it impacting negatively on his enjoyment of play, then it is something I would work on a little more. I do think that your son has picked up on your anxieties around mess – unfortunately, this is very common. When we start feeding babies we pass on our own feelings by being a little too eager to wipe away food from their faces and hands and, as you quite rightly point out, this can send messages that can negatively impact on them as they grow. We also need to be concerned about our language. If you tend to call things 'mucky', 'dirty', 'messy' or 'yucky', there is a good chance that your son is picking up on these negative words and associating them with different textures. This needn't be just food-related; it can also be associated with play – for instance, if you say, 'Mind the yucky mud, you don't want to get dirty'. So as well as being mindful of your own actions, being mindful of your language is equally important.

I think you're doing the right thing by encouraging exploration with different textures through play. This doesn't have to be 'messy play' per se, though. Natural ways to introduce children to different textures through everyday life include encouraging him to dig in the garden with you and touch mud while you are planting or weeding, helping you to prepare food for dinner, especially different vegetables, and helping to bake – kneading dough works particularly well. When you do this, be sure to use positive language to describe the textures he is exposed to. I would also look to children's books or even television programmes that involve positive sensory play – Peppa Pig jumping in muddy puddles, for example, and the characters eating different foods, including vegetables. Hopefully, your son's sensory aversions, particularly surrounding food, will fade as he grows. However, there is a possibility that he could have sensory processing disorder, which can cause children to struggle with certain textures and sensory stimulation, so that they may actively avoid some exposures. This can impact on everything from their play to the clothes they wear and the food that they eat. If you do feel concerned about your son's sensory issues, then I would recommend booking an appointment with your GP for investigation and, most importantly, some specialist therapy, which could make a big difference to your son.

The second aspect to consider involves the boundaries you have in place surrounding eating and particularly your son's television viewing. While I completely understand that you have set a boundary around television, my advice would be to completely separate this from his eating. Your attempts to negotiate with your son to eat a few more spoonsful in order to be able to watch television could have a negative impact on his eating behaviour in later life. Essentially, what you are doing here is encouraging your child to ignore and override his own bodily signals concerning his hunger and satiety. As the television is such a draw for him, he is likely to follow your command to eat a little more because he knows he will then get what he wants – the television. Unfortunately, this teaches him that if he eats more, he gets something pleasurable; he is learning to eat more than he needs and to ignore the cues his body is giving him to stop. There is a chance that this may lead to overeating and even obesity as he grows, as he becomes less and less able to listen to his body's cues and continues to eat, even when he is not hungry, especially as there is an emotional element of pleasure following the eating. I would recommend that you reconsider your television boundaries and make them entirely independent of food. For instance, you could allow only one hour per day, first thing in the morning, or one hour per day in the afternoon, well away from food. I also recommend that you try to never prompt your son to eat. Prompting children to eat is strongly associated with overeating and an increased obesity risk and doesn't improve what they eat in the short term.

Q. *Our son is currently two years and three months old. As he soon as he wakes, he screams for his bottle. If he sees another child eating, he demands snacks. Picnics with friends and meals out are a nightmare, as he just wants food all the time if he sees it and won't stop eating. Other children seem to just have the odd snack and lose interest, but he finishes them all. We don't let him have any junk food and are careful with portion sizes, as we always need to consider that he will finish everything he is given. One theory we have is that he uses food as a comfort, to help himself navigate the day, as he asks for snacks more when friends come around and he is unsettled. We would really value your views on how we can help manage his eating better.*

A. It is entirely possible that your son's eating is normal. Some toddlers barely eat anything and some eat all day. I have had one of each! While picky eating is standard in toddlerhood, that doesn't mean non-picky eating isn't. I think the most important thing to consider here is whether your son is otherwise healthy and an appropriate height and weight for his age. This doesn't mean that he should be of *average* height and weight; it's OK if he is bigger than average, so long as his height and weight are in proportion.

We do know that babies who are bottle-fed are more at risk of overeating than those who are exclusively breastfed, largely because it is possible to overfeed a baby with a bottle because it is harder for them to regulate their own satiety, or feelings of fullness. (With a bottle, the baby is in less control than they would be if they were breastfed.) I do think it is worth keeping this in mind. Similarly, you could be correct in your assumption that food is being used as a comfort measure. Here, I would be very careful that you never use food of any form as a reward, be it for 'good behaviour' or even in potty training. You also need to be very careful that you don't use food as a form of distraction, to avoid having to cope with tantrums or other difficult behaviour. And, finally, you should never use food as a way to cheer him up. The same also applies to your own eating. You are an incredibly powerful role model and if your son sees or hears you referring to food as a palliative for uncomfortable emotions – such as anger, sadness, boredom or stress – he will quickly learn to copy you.

What you need to do is to completely separate food from emotions. If you see your son feeling anxious, stressed or sad, don't be afraid to sit with his tears and frustration. Make sure you always give him the impression that it's OK for him to express his emotions with you, no matter how loud, difficult or embarrassing they may be. If you know he is asking for food to cope with his emotions, I would instead give him a big hug, sit with him and encourage him to talk about how he is feeling. Initially, this is likely to make him really unsettled as he's used to getting food but, in a way, this is good, as it helps him to release all the feelings that he has been keeping inside.

Next, I strongly recommend that you try to drop as much control surrounding your son's eating as possible. Scientific research shows that the more parents try to control their children's eating, the more likely they are to overeat and eat in secret. Your goal is to help your son to recognise true feelings of hunger and satiety and to eat only when he is hungry and stop when he is full. Related to this, I suggest that you stop restricting your son, whether that is prohibiting 'junk food' or limiting portion sizes. This tends to be viewed as deprivation.

And what do we want most when we feel deprived of something? We want that something a lot more. If you restrict certain foods now, junk or otherwise, you are creating a very real risk that your son will binge on them as soon as he has access to them. This is the very same reason why diets not only don't work, but make people put on weight. Although it may seem entirely counterproductive, you really want your son to feel that he can have the food he wants, when he wants it. Of course, I'm not saying you should fill your house with junk food, but just consider loosening the reins a little. And in terms of portion sizes, this is one area that your son really needs to control himself. I recommend that you don't serve him food, but instead place it in serving dishes and give your son an empty plate. Encourage him to serve himself – he may need a little help with the physicality of this since he is only two, but as much as possible, let him be in control. Allow him to put on his plate only what he feels he is hungry for, and remind him that if he is still hungry when he has finished he can return and serve himself more. The first few times he does this, don't be surprised if he has not only second, but third, fourth and fifth helpings. This novelty should soon wear off and you should find he begins to eat less.

You could also try having a grazing tray – a tray or plate with different sections, containing a variety of foods that you prepare and leave out for him. The tray should be placed where he can access it easily himself, returning to it to take whatever he likes, whenever he wants to. Again, I understand this may seem counterproductive and, initially, he will probably eat even more food than usual. However, ultimately, with food always available, he should begin to feel safer in the knowledge that he won't be deprived if he is genuinely hungry. And when the novelty of free access to food wears off, you should find that he actually eats less of it.

Finally, I would encourage your son to move as much

as possible. Lots of running around outside, visiting parks, kicking balls around, climbing, dancing and running. Make sure movement is a joy, not a chore, which it almost always is to a toddler.

The toddler and preschooler years are possibly the most frustrating and yet fulfilling years of parenthood. Following the principles of gentle eating – staying mindful, empowering your child, remaining respectful of them and approaching feeding in an authoritative and responsive way – will, hopefully, remove a great deal of the frustration that surrounds the typical eating habits of young children, leaving you free to enjoy the crazy, happy and fulfilling ride.

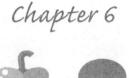

Chapter 6

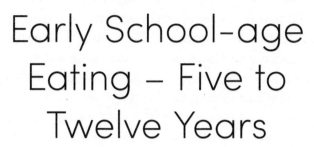

Early School-age Eating – Five to Twelve Years

For the first four years of a child's life, their parents hold almost all the influence over their eating. When they start school, however, this is rapidly redistributed. Friends, teachers and education policymakers all impact on not only how a child eats, but how they think about eating. Some of this influence is positive, some less so – and the latter can open the doors to a whole new raft of eating issues that most likely have never been encountered by families before. My aim with this chapter is to introduce you to the most common eating hurdles faced during the early school years and, importantly, to consider how to overcome them, in a gentle and effective manner.

Eating and education – clashes and control

The tenets of gentle eating – being mindful, empowering, respectful and authoritative – are never tested more in childhood than when a child starts school. No matter how much schools try to improve the health of students through the implementation of healthy-eating policies, education and awareness, their efforts sadly almost always fall into the authoritarian camp.

Authoritarian control of eating means just that: control – whether that is asserted through school rules, food monitoring, weight checks or attempting to change eating habits through fear. Ironically, an authoritarian approach to eating will nearly always backfire. Even if attempts at controlling students' eating are successful in the short term, the chances are that the long term will bring negative and unintended consequences, with a significantly greater risk of obesity.[1] Sadly, even the most well-intentioned eating interventions employed by schools carry a very real risk to the eating habits and beliefs of children and, in their efforts to improve things, schools often make them far worse. Let's look at a few of the issues in a little more detail.

Regimented eating times

Gentle-eating principles focus on helping children to follow their body's hunger and satiety signals, so that they will respond to feelings of hunger by eating and then stop when they feel full. Over the last three chapters I have highlighted the importance of trusting a child when they say that they are hungry, or full, by not forcing them to eat and not doubting them when they say that they are hungry. This respect empowers children and allows them to form a positive relationship with food that will last throughout their lives. Unfortunately, when children start school, they can no longer eat when they are hungry or, indeed, not eat when they are not. They are expected to eat only when the school says they can. This means that they must learn to override their feelings of hunger during lesson times, when it is deemed inappropriate for them to eat, and they must eat at lunchtime, even if they are not hungry. This goes back to the idea we discussed in Chapter 1 – that is, eating at times when it is socially accepted (breakfast, lunch and dinner), rather than when your body tells you to. The time between starting and leaving school and lunchtime may be short, but for a child who is otherwise used to eating 'on demand', even a few hours can be problematic.

Packed-lunch policies

Lunch itself can put immense pressure on children. Many schools now have packed-lunch policies. These prohibit choco-late, crisps, soft drinks and anything else the school deems to be unhealthy. At first, this might seem like a good idea, especially when research has found that the nutritional content of packed lunches is significantly poorer than that of school dinners.[2] Packed lunches tend to be higher in calories, sugar and sodium than the food served by schools. These policies do, however, have a much darker side. They can encourage feelings of guilt, secrecy and shame when children try to sneak contraband in and especially when they get caught for it and their food is con-fiscated. Naively, it is often believed that such policies will result in healthier choices and reduce the amount of 'unhealthy food' eaten by children; but, in reality, it simply means that the child will fill up on it when they get home from school, leading to secret eating and bingeing, which is characteristic of disordered eating. So while these measures are put in place with the well-being of the children in mind, they often create far greater problems than those they seek to resolve. Perhaps this risk would be worth taking if they had a positive impact on a significant number of children. Sadly, they don't. Research has shown that food and drink policies at school have limited results in tackling obesity and food choices.[3] They are simply not anywhere near as successful as many schools seem to believe.

School dinners

While headway has been made in terms of the nutritional content of school meals in recent years, they are not without problems. Policing of school dinners still exists. Dinner ladies will commonly stop children from ordering what they want to eat, portion sizes are not controlled by children, desserts are still held as the holy grail and only given once children have eaten 'enough' of their main meal. And the desserts themselves are often far more energy dense than a child would eat if left to their own devices. One of the biggest issues with school meals, however, is the very short time allocated for children to eat them. The average school lunch hour is precisely that – an hour long. In this hour, children need to eat, visit the toilet and play. Often, school meals are split into separate shifts if the whole school cannot fit into the hall or cafeteria at once and naturally staff are anxious to move children along, so that the next shift can eat. Research has shown that children have, on average, only seven minutes to eat their lunch at school.[4] What happens when they have insufficient time? They compensate by speeding up their eating. This increased speed and the lack of control over eating can result in them overriding their satiety levels and overeating, which completely negates any of the positives surrounding school meals.

Rewarding eating

Praise and reward for eating are rife in many schools, with adults saying, 'Well done!' when children try something new or eat all their lunch. When they were younger, my children often came home from school with stickers or certificates given for 'good eating'. While some school staff may realise that rewarding a child for clearing their plate may not be such a good idea, they might think that praising them for trying something new is sensible. The simple fact is, rewards and praise in any form are a bad idea when it comes to eating. School staff should try as hard as possible to remain neutral and not comment on what children are (or are not) eating. Most importantly, the stickers and certificates with smiley faces and stars proclaiming, 'I ate all my lunch today' really need to go.

Healthy-eating education

As childhood obesity levels rise, there seem to be more and more governmental schemes attempting to reverse the trend. The schemes are well-intentioned (albeit not entirely aimed at helping children – after all, the less obesity there is, the less money the government needs to spend on obesity-related healthcare), but they generally fall wide of the mark. In the last couple of years, I have noticed that schools' involvement in 'healthy-eating education' has cranked up several gears, with healthy-eating weeks, workshops and handouts now commonplace and undoubtedly set to increase as efforts fail and childhood obesity trends continue to rise.

Classroom-based 'healthy-eating awareness' is not what is needed to make a positive change. At best, it teaches children what they hopefully already know and, at worst, it makes them feel guilty, shamed, inadequate and, perhaps, a little obsessive about their eating. And what do these feelings lead to? Far from the healthy changes the policymakers and course writers hope to achieve, they are more likely to lead children to eat in secret, overly control their eating – giving rise to orthorexia (see page 38) – and then, ultimately, binge when they feel that they have failed.

But school efforts to influence eating are not the only problem. Attempts to control children's movement also have negative consequences that can last way beyond their school years, contributing, again, to the obesity that exercise in school aims to beat.

Exercise as a lesson

Before they start school, children move for fun. They run, skip, jump, roll, climb, dance and hop for no reason other than it feels good to do so. For young children, moving and playing are one and the same. But when school starts, movement becomes a lesson, like any other subject. PE lessons attempt to control how children move their bodies in order to teach them how to do it better. 'Mile-a-day' initiatives (where children run for the first ten minutes of every school day) are meant to keep children fit and help them to focus, but what they really do is to control how, how much and when children move each day. And the moment something becomes academic, it no longer feels natural to children. Moving their own bodies becomes something that they are not fully in control of.

What happens when children are not good at PE? I was one of those children. Before I started school, I loved to spend hours dancing around my house, my beloved skipping rope was my favourite toy and I loved to swim. Once I started school, however, I soon realised that I was not good at rope climbing, I was clumsy at running and my swimming was slow. PE lessons undermined my love of moving; they turned it into a chore – and chores were not something I wanted to repeat at home.

Recently, my daughter's school held a healthy-eating week. We were asked to send our children to school dressed in 'sporty attire' so that they could take part in a week of sports activities. As I dropped her off on the first day, I felt a pang of sorrow for the bigger, less fit children in the school, squeezed into ill-fitting tracksuits, knowing that they were going to spend a week feeling inadequate and useless – that when they couldn't do something their peers could do, they would feel shamed and guilty, despite the teachers' talk of growth mindsets and cheers of encouragement. I knew that when they got home at the end of the day they would be tempted to drown their sorrows in bars of chocolate or packets of crisps, but would feel even more awful knowing that they were failing at being healthy. At some point, the fall would come and when it hit, it would hit hard. I know the week was arranged with good intentions, but forcing children to exercise, especially for a whole week, is not the way to make them love moving their bodies again. Children need less of that pressure, not more.

Restricting movement in class

If parents have an issue with their child's movement before they start school, it is usually that their child moves too much, not too little. But once school starts, children's movement is automatically restricted. During the average six-and-a-half-hour school day, they spend only one and a half hours moving – that's twenty-five hours fewer per week than before they started school. This huge reduction in movement is problematic. Not only does it undoubtedly influence fitness and weight, it also negatively affects children's learning. Schools must find a way to encourage children to move more, throughout the whole school day, not just during break times and PE lessons.

Restricting movement as a discipline tool

As if spending five hours per day unable to move much isn't bad enough, many schools utilise break and lunchtimes for children to catch up on work, or as a form of discipline. Lunchtime detentions are commonly used in secondary or high schools, and even in some primary schools too, albeit usually by another name. Of course, forcing more physical inactivity on children by 'keeping them behind' to manage poor behaviour, while their peers are allowed out into the playground, will only make them struggle with inactivity even more in class. Despite research showing the problems with restricting break times, and professional organisations warning against it (in 2012 the American Academy of Pediatrics advised recess 'should not be withheld for punitive or academic reasons'), it continues to be used as a common discipline tool.[5]

What can schools do?

In spite of their best efforts, most schools currently do more harm than good when it comes to increasing healthy eating and reducing obesity. But does this mean there is nothing that they can do to effect a positive change? In fact, there are several ways in which schools can help, but their approach needs to radically change. In short, the best line schools can take when it comes to eating is to adopt gentle-eating principles. How would that look in practice?

- **Mindful** Provide opportunities for children to focus on their eating, without feeling rushed to attend a lunchtime detention or squeeze some play into a day otherwise dominated by sitting still.

- **Empowering** Help children to enjoy eating and moving, by encouraging them to realise that both are enjoyable and rewarding, not a chore or something to worry too much about. Involve children in the whole process, from understanding how their bodies work to how food is produced. Help them to develop the skills they need to eat well for the rest of their lives, not just lecture them about 'healthy eating'.

- **Respectful** Avoid praising or rewarding children's eating, prompting them to eat more or to try something new and respecting their individual hunger and satiety signals, likes and dislikes.

- **Authoritative** Drop the control. Remove lunchbox policing and school-dinner rules. Allow children to eat what they want, without shame or guilt and especially without pressure to eat something the school considers healthier. Give children different opportunities to move, instead of forcing them to take part in a particular sporting activity if it is not something that they enjoy.

There are three, very specific, school-based activities that have been shown repeatedly to make a positive and long-lasting change to children's eating. Interestingly, each involves the child being fully immersed in a multi-sensory experience, not in a classroom listening to a talk or a workshop about food, weight or exercise, or seated in front of a computer learning about 'healthy eating'. Children learn best by doing – something known as experiential learning, when the subject matter sparks their imagination and, most importantly, when they enjoy what they're doing. It may not surprise you, therefore, that the activities which can really help are gardening, cooking and shopping.

Sadly, with the ever-increasing pressure on schools to meet higher and higher academic standards, there is little time to focus on the subjects deemed 'less important'. In fact, those that are most helpful in terms of developing a healthy relationship with food are the ones that children are least likely to do, although it is not hard to weave them into the school syllabus, and they can be used to support the national curriculum with their applicability to science and mathematics. Similarly, they don't call for a huge amount of extra space (gardening can easily be done in small pots outside classrooms) or expenditure. In my local school, parents donate seeds, compost, pots and cookery equipment and ingredients, and help to run special sessions and clubs. They are all doable, in all settings, with enough planning.

Growing food

Research into the eating habits of six- and seven-year-olds found that when they took part in school gardening classes this resulted in superior knowledge and increased liking and consumption of fruit and vegetables when compared with their peers who had classroom-based nutritional education sessions.[6] Growing food gives children ownership and control. They can choose the varieties of fruit and vegetables to plant, select the seeds and the areas in which to plant them. After planting, they can be responsible for watering and feeding the seedlings, weeding the area, supporting stems and, finally, harvesting the resulting crop. This whole process gives them far better knowledge than they would ever gain in the classroom, the familiarity of the plants helps to reduce neophobia (see page 111) and picky eating and the sense of ownership and pride acts as a motivator for them to eat their produce, rather than just being told that they should eat certain foods because they are healthy. The positive effects of growing food are not just restricted to school; it works equally well at home. You don't need any special equipment or lots of space – just a couple of small tubs or pots on a windowsill can be enough to accommodate an impressive crop.

Cooking food

The logical follow on from growing food is cooking it. Once again, research has shown that getting hands-on with food during cookery lessons at school results in better outcomes than classroom-based education.[7] These outcomes are better still if the children have also been involved in growing the ingredients that they are cooking with. Cooking helps children on a sensory level, so that they become familiarised with foods through touch, sight and smell, as well as taste; plus, the hands-on involvement can help to reduce picky eating and neophobia. Learning to cook is one of the most important skills to teach children. While they may not need to know algebra as adults or remember what they learned about the First World War in school, they will use the skills gained in cookery classes daily. But teaching children how to cook is not something that should be reserved for school – as parents, it is one of the most valuable ways in which you can spend your time if you are concerned about their eating.

Shopping for food

If children aren't growing the food that they eat, the next best thing is involving them in shopping for it, ideally at a farmers' market. By meeting the farmers, children can feel more involved in the history of the food that they will be consuming, and helping to select the food they will eat gives them a degree of control that they don't ordinarily have. With their large halls and good outside space, schools provide a perfect location for local farmers' markets, and bringing the sale of food to the children – perhaps immediately after school, or at a weekend, when parents can be present to buy – empowers them to shop for the food that they will eat. Research considering the impact of school-based farmers' markets has found that they result in an improved attitude towards food in children, as well as an increased consumption of fruit and vegetables,[8] which would surely be compounded if the children were then involved in the preparation of that food as well.

If your child's school is unable or reluctant to introduce these measures, a good option is to meet with the PTA (parent-teacher association) to discuss the idea of parents running an after-school club to take up these activities. At my daughter's school, parents run a very busy and successful gardening and cookery club each week.

Sticks and stones, weight and teasing

There are several things schools can do to improve the messages they give to children concerning health and eating, and parents can help in the development of healthier policies. What schools and parents will always struggle to control, however, is the impact of other children. Teasing and bullying about weight have always existed, and their impact is far greater than most people realise. Even if you don't believe that your child is being teased, or is indeed teasing others, it is still important to understand the implications because we never quite know everything that is happening in the lives of our children.

Weight-related teasing is an unfortunate reality for many

children, with school being the most common place for it to occur, across all ages. It affects both girls and boys, with over-weight girls being four times more likely to be teased by their peers than boys,[9] while overweight boys who are teased are alarmingly far more likely to become bullies themselves than their non-overweight peers.[10] Children who are teased about their weight are also more likely to be excluded by their peers, both in class and in the playground.[11]

We must ask the question, are these children the target of teasing solely because of their weight, or is the excess weight a symptom of a social or emotional issue that causes them to struggle to interact with their peers – something that would still exist (and perhaps be the target of teasing) even if they were not overweight. If so, this would mean that these children are hyper-vulnerable to bullying and friendship issues. Research has shown that children who are teased by their peers are more likely to struggle with emotional eating,[12] which makes sense – because when children feel sad and hurt by the teasing, they turn to the one thing that they know will temporarily make them feel better: food. Children who are teased by their peers for their weight are also considerably more likely to be depressed[13] and perform significantly worse than their peers academically too.[14] And the effects of being teased about weight in childhood unfortunately don't dissipate in adulthood either. Research has found that adults who were teased for their weight as children are appreciably more likely to have disturbed eating behaviours than their peers who were not.[15]

Teasing has serious and long-lasting effects and is not some-thing that can be ignored. It is not enough to talk to your child about the teasing and tell them to ignore it. Sticks and stones hurt, but so do words – perhaps even more so. The teasing must be stopped. To facilitate this, you must foster a relationship with your child that enables them to talk to you about anything. This means listening quietly and earnestly and not replying with stock phrases such as, 'Don't be silly, just ignore them'. Explain to your child that you want to help, that they shouldn't have to put up with the teasing and that you will speak to their teachers. It is important that your child has faith that you can help them.

Keep a written record of the teasing, making a note of when it happened, who was involved and what was said, as well as any adults your child spoke to about it. Next, request a meeting with your child's form teacher to discuss the teasing and ask them what they plan to do to resolve the problem. If this does not achieve results, your next step is to request a meeting with the school head or principal. If this meeting again is unsatisfactory, then your next step is to make a complaint to the school's board of governors. Take notes at all meetings and keep them safe, along with any correspondence. The school has a duty to resolve your issue. If, after you've taken all the above steps, it still fails to do so, then sadly, your only alternative may be to look for a new school.

What should you do if you find that your own child is teasing others because of their weight? First, you must ascertain whether *they* are being bullied. Bullies are often bullied themselves. If this is the case, you must work with them to stop it; hopefully, once the cause has been removed, the symptoms will naturally disappear. If your child isn't being bullied, then your role is to help them to understand how their teasing makes others feel. Young children do not have especially advanced empathy skills and often don't realise the impact of their behaviour. You may find that an online video explaining bullying from the perspective of the victim works much better than just a conversation. Alternatively, a simple and striking visual way to explain the effects of bullying is to get a piece of paper and screw it up. Tell your child: 'This is me bullying the paper. Can you see I have hurt it by screwing it up?' Next, say to your child, 'Now, I'm going to stop being mean to the paper. I'm going to open it up and smooth it out. This is me saying, "I'm sorry".' Open the paper and show it to your child. Ask them, 'Does the paper look the same to you? Or does it look different from how it did before I screwed it up? Can you see all the lines and creases? That's what bullying does. It doesn't matter if you're sorry and apologise. It doesn't make the pain go away. There are always lasting marks.' Tell them that teasing hurts. Everybody has feelings and teasing may cause permanent damage if it continues. This works really well for children of all ages.

Changes in body image and confidence

Shocking research shows that girls start to have concerns about their bodies and begin dieting as young as six years of age, with awareness and consideration of dieting increasing with age.[16] Interviews with girls aged six and seven found that they rated their ideal figure as significantly thinner than their current frame. As children approach puberty, it is natural that they become more conscious of their bodies. However, for some, particularly girls, this is a dangerous time. Girls who perceived themselves as overweight before puberty began, even if they weren't, showed significantly worse body image and disordered eating than those who did not.[17] While boys are not immune from the emotional effects of puberty and body-image issues, girls are significantly more likely to struggle and experience disordered eating and eating disorders as a result. When asking why this is, we cannot ignore the impact of the media and advertising. Young girls today are exposed to increasingly unrealistic portrayals of body shapes and sizes, from the non-existent waists and hips of the dolls they play with to the overtly sexual clothing of underweight young female pop singers. Pictures and stories in magazines intended for pre-teen girls bombard them with imagery and ideas that undoubtedly give rise to body anxiety and unacceptance. Research into 300 six- to nine-year-old girls found that this exposure to sexualised media correlated with girls internalising sexualised messages, which, in turn, caused them to be more likely to develop a negative body image.[18] Girls today are faced with more of these inappropriate images and messages than any generation in the past. It is a ticking time bomb. If we want our girls to grow up to feel good about themselves, and have a positive relationship with their bodies and with eating, we must do something – and quickly.

Raising girls with a positive body image

The first thing to do is to try to lessen the negative impact of the media on children by reducing exposure as much as possible. This means avoiding the magazines and videos that portray unrealistic ideals, monitoring Internet usage and restricting access to social-media channels, in particular until the teen years.

Next, arguably the most important influence on young girls when it comes to body image and eating habits is their mother. Research has found that a mother's behaviour and her feelings about her own body have a direct impact on her daughter's body image and dieting behaviour.[19] In Chapter 2, I outlined the importance of exorcising your own eating demons, so as not to pass on your beliefs to your children. This is even more important if you have a daughter. To raise a daughter with a healthy body image, you must work on your own, avoiding dieting and making sure that the messages you are giving out are positive (see the table about positive body talk on page 34).

There are several other ways in which you can increase the chances that your daughter will feel good about herself and reduce the likelihood that she will develop disordered eating:

- Do you comment when you see somebody who is particularly large or skinny? Or do you praise others for their weight loss? Be mindful of how you speak about others and avoid commenting on their bodies.

- Avoid praising your daughter for her looks. Compliment her on what she does and what she achieves in life, not what she looks like.

- Help your daughter to understand puberty and what is, or will be, happening to her, preferably well in advance of it starting. Help her to frame puberty and the impending changes to her body in a positive way and be open and honest with her, so she feels able to ask you anything. I began speaking to my own daughter about puberty when she was seven, in order that she would be well prepared and relaxed when it started to happen.

- Implement a way of communicating in writing, so she can ask you questions she may be too shy to ask face to face. My daughter and I had a journal we could both write in, exchanging personal and potentially embarrassing messages to each other.

- Expose your daughter to good examples of positive body image. Think about the messages in the television programmes, films or online videos she watches and in the books that she reads. Try to find a heroine for her to look up to.

- Help your daughter to spot unrealistic portrayals of female bodies. Look at images together and watch videos about photoshop manipulation.

- Choose dolls with realistic body shapes. This means the most popular dolls are out, unfortunately – Barbie and Bratz, in particular.

- Avoid cosmetics and beauty products targeted at children and ask friends and relatives not to purchase them for your daughter as presents.

- Choose clothes for little girls, not mini women. Try to find retailers that sell roomy clothes, not skimpily cut ones, and talk about the comfort and practicalities of clothing, rather than the aesthetics.

- Choose books with powerful female role models, in which girls are portrayed as capable, strong, clever and funny, rather than just pretty and popular (see 'Girls and positive body image' in Useful Resources, page 206).

- Encourage a hobby, especially one that involves regularly meeting with their peers, such as Guiding, or playing a musical instrument in a band.

- Find a way in which your daughter can enjoy moving her body – for instance cycling, swimming, climbing or dancing. Place the emphasis on how much fun and how healthy it is to move and how strong her body is, rather than on how she looks.

- Focus on gratitude. Help your daughter to recognise how lucky she is to have a strong and healthy body.

While there is no denying that the pre-teen years can be significantly harder for girls than they are for boys, the above also applies to those raising sons, particularly if they are having doubts over their bodies and their self-worth based on their looks.

When your child is overweight

Children are significantly more likely to become overweight as they approach the teen years. Obesity levels in the UK rise sharply from 9 per cent at age five to 19 per cent at age eleven. Diagnosis of obesity is controversial sometimes, though, especially when it comes from school weight monitoring.

School weight-monitoring schemes focus on children's body mass index (BMI) – a measurement that calculates ideal weight based on height. However, this may not be the best way to diagnose obesity in children, despite the fact that it is commonly used.[20] It takes no account of an individual child's build or muscle mass. It also ignores something known as 'central adiposity', or fat carried around the tummy and hips, which has a significantly more important impact on the child's future health than that distributed more evenly over the body.

But while school weight monitoring may be unreliable because of the focus on BMI, research finds that parents often don't admit their child has a weight problem when they do.[21] If you do feel that your child is overweight, what should you do – or perhaps, more importantly, not do? Let's start with what you shouldn't do.

As we have already seen several times, scientists have consistently found that if parents attempt to control their children's eating, taking an authoritarian approach, they are more likely to be overweight.[22] The same applies when children are overweight and parents are seeking ways to help them lose weight. The more you try to control their eating, the more likely they are to gain weight, not lose it, and develop eating problems for the rest of their lives. Research looking at children between five and seven years of age has found that when parents place firmer limits on eating, children are more likely to eat in the absence of hunger.[23] In other words, restricting food, or placing a child on a diet, has the reverse effect to that intended, making them eat more and override their satiety signals. Further research shows that when parents prohibit their children from eating snacks, they eat significantly more and, importantly, they desire the banned food much more than children who are not restricted.[24] Putting your child on a diet is a very strong 'no no', according to science.

Does this mean that you should just ignore your child's weight? There is an argument for this. Not making an issue of it is perhaps the healthiest way to help them to regain control of their eating habits. And the principles of gentle eating once again apply here:

- Help your child to be mindful of their eating – to understand the difference between hunger and appetite – encouraging them to be aware of their body's signs of satiety.

- Respect that they are able to recognise these cues in their own bodies and the choices they make when following them. Reduce distractions around eating and place boundaries on where it happens – never in front of a screen, for instance. Help your child to develop non-food-related strategies to cope with their emotions, such as downloading a mindfulness relaxation recording for children or buying them a stress ball to squeeze when they feel anxious or angry. Once again, focusing on developing a positive body image is key. Help your child to realise that they are not their weight and should never define themselves by it.

- Keep a check on your parenting, making sure that your approach to your child's eating is authoritative and not authoritarian and try to resist stepping in and taking control or placing limits on what your child eats.

- Finally, empower your child to enjoy moving their body again, just as they did in early childhood. Find something that your child enjoys and place the emphasis on just that: enjoyment – not getting fit or losing weight. Taking part in an activity with them can turn it into something far more fun, such as going on a family bike ride, hiring a badminton court for the whole family at your local leisure centre every weekend or going on a hike together for the day. These family activities will have benefits over and above the movement and exercise, bringing you closer together and enabling your child to open up to you more about their anxieties and concerns, which, in turn, will reduce their need for emotional eating.

When your child is underweight

While obesity and overweight are the most significant weight concerns in school-age children, some do struggle with being underweight, and picky eating often remains a challenge throughout childhood. Parenting an underweight child can be just as hard as parenting one who is overweight, and despite their seeming like very different problems, the advice remains very similar if there is no underlying medical issue.

Once again, gentle-eating principles top the list of advice:

- Empower your child to be mindful about their eating, particularly paying attention to their hunger cues and not missing them because of distractions.

- Allow your child to take some control over their eating, approaching food in an authoritative, not authoritarian manner.

- Respect that your child's choices are in order.

If your child remains a picky eater, then the advice is the same as coping with picky eating in toddlerhood and the preschool years. Familiarise them with different foods with repeated exposure, involving them in growing, choosing, preparing and cooking meals with you. Take any pressure away: don't force your child to eat, reward or praise them for eating and, especially, don't admonish them for not eating. Trust your child to follow their own bodily cues and accept their likes and dislikes by giving them control over what they eat. Following these steps may not produce fast results, but they will, ultimately, lead to the healthiest outcome for your child. In the meantime, you may consider a good-quality vitamin and mineral supplement if you feel that your child is not getting enough nutrition from their diet.

Most children who are underweight are entirely healthy and their weight may be something that will gradually change over time, although some will stay slight for their whole life – again, not everybody is average, and it's OK for some to be smaller than others. A small minority of underweight children do, however, have an underlying medical condition. As a parent, your instinct is valuable here. If you intuitively feel that something is wrong and there is a reason for your child's low weight, trust yourself and push for investigation with your family doctor. My firstborn, the one-time picky eater, suddenly became very underweight after starting school, despite overcoming his pickiness and starting school at a healthy weight. Alongside his weight loss he seemed lethargic and would regularly complain about being tired and unable to walk. I knew something was wrong, but our GP dismissed my worries, saying that he seemed OK, just on the slight side, and was probably tired from starting school. I persisted until she ordered blood tests. A week later I received a phone call to say that the blood results were back and I needed to return to the surgery with my son. The first thing our GP did when I walked in the room was to apologise for not taking my concerns seriously. My son's blood test results had come back positive for coeliac disease, later confirmed by a biopsy. Coeliac disease is an autoimmune condition in which the consumption of gluten causes an immune response in the body and an inability to absorb important nutrients, causing malnutrition. The treatment is a lifelong gluten-free diet. Coeliac UK estimate that one in 100 people is affected, yet only one in four is currently diagnosed. My son is now a big, strapping teenager, but back then something inside me kept telling me that his weight was not normal. If you feel that your child may have an underlying problem, please do seek medical advice.

Allergies and special eating needs

When a child is younger, handling food allergies and intolerances is relatively simple. But when they reach school age, you not only have to trust others to follow instructions to keep them safe, you also need to trust the child themselves to not eat something they shouldn't. My biggest worry when my son was diagnosed with coeliac disease, however, was how he would cope emotionally with the restrictions on his eating and the differences between him and his peers.

Children with coeliac disease are at significantly greater risk of developing anxiety and eating disorders than their non-coeliac peers.[25] While it is possible that there is a physiological cause for this, sharing an aetiology with the disease itself, it is impossible to discard the emotional effects of living with a condition that exerts a significant amount of control over which foods are eaten, especially when you consider the implications of feeling socially excluded. Parties, visits to friends' houses, school trips and special events suddenly presented hurdles that we had never appreciated before. This is true for parents of children not only with coeliac disease, but those with food allergies too.

In our case, my son's school was ill equipped to handle his eating needs, and so he was unable to eat school meals. On a day-to-day basis this was not an issue, since he preferred packed lunches, but it meant he missed out on special meals, such as Christmas lunch. I quickly learned that the best way to help him to feel normal was to provide him with 'safe' food myself. I made him a special Christmas packed lunch, complete with a Christmas cracker, to take to school, and I would send him to parties with a selection of gluten-free party food. Alongside this, we joined our local coeliac support group and attended monthly meetings, which helped to normalise his disease and eating needs. Meeting other coeliacs and exchanging food tips was an important part of his acceptance of his eating needs. Finally, I spent a lot of time helping him to understand what was happening inside his body, why his needs were different and what would happen if he did eat gluten.

Now, as a teenager, he has full control of his diet and I have told him that it is his decision if he chooses to eat gluten and that I trust him. To date, he has never purposefully eaten food containing gluten – something his consultant gastroenterologist is continually surprised by, as teenage coeliacs usually 'fall off the wagon' after all the years of parental control in childhood.

In conclusion, I firmly believe that the best way to handle special eating needs is to help the child to feel in control and as normal as possible.

Candy chaos

Sugar is possibly the hottest topic in nutrition now. It is hard to escape any discussion about it, especially when related to childhood obesity.

A growing number of parents attempt to avoid processed sugar in their children's diets and some prohibit all sweets and chocolate completely. Despite this, research shows that children eat significantly more sugar in their school years than compared with toddlers and preschoolers.[26] Sugar consumption also declines as they enter adulthood. So the two questions immediately raised by these findings are what causes the increase in sugar consumption and what can parents do about it? The answer to both questions is one and the same: it is highly likely that the sharp increase in sugar consumption in school-age children is, at least in part, due to its restriction by parents. The way to reduce the sugar obsession? Drop the restrictions and remove the control around its consumption.

Most parents look at me in horror when I suggest this to them. Nevertheless, relinquishing control is almost always the best way to handle sugar, sweets and chocolate. Research has shown that limiting sweets and chocolate has negative consequences, including the development of an increased desire for them, more attention being focused on trying to obtain them and a tendency to overeat them when the restrictions are removed.[27] Simply, if we want children to be able to control their sugar consumption, we must let them eat it and trust that they will self-regulate. Parental eating habits are important here. If you, as an adult, view cakes, biscuits, chocolate and sweets as 'special', eating them as a 'treat', limiting them and referring to them as 'naughty', then you model this belief to your children and they will not be able to self-regulate their consumption either.

Children need to view all sources of food equally. To eat instinctively, in line with their hunger and satiety levels, children must be allowed to choose what they eat. The minute we impose restrictions, we remove their ability to self-regulate.

What should you do if you are already restricting sugar? My firm opinion is that you should relinquish control. The more you restrict, the more difficult it will be for your child to self-regulate when they do eventually eat the 'forbidden fruit'. This, I believe, is why children eat significantly more sugar when they are of school age: what happens when their parents are not around to control their food choices? Of course, they are finally free to choose what they want, and previously forbidden foods are the most appealing. I was raised in a house where pudding was only ever fruit. Cake was for birthdays and Christmas only and chocolate and sweets were banned, as were sugary drinks. It is no surprise, then, that the moment I was away from my mother, I gorged on all things sugary. I sneaked them into our house and ate them in my bedroom in secret. Sugar became my guilty secret – and guilty secrets are incredibly powerful, especially when they lead to feelings of self-reproach and emotional eating as a result. My mother's motives were well-intentioned. She wanted me to develop healthy eating habits and a stable, healthy weight. Sadly, however, by not keeping sugary foods in the house and restricting them throughout my childhood, the result was the opposite of what she'd intended.

I have tried hard to not limit sugar for my own children, in order that they grow up with the ability to self-regulate, unlike me. Despite the very mindful and informed choice behind my actions, I am still astounded when we go grocery shopping and they ask if they can choose something to eat, returning with a banana, some grapes or a bread roll, instead of the chocolate or cake that would always tempt me.

Questions from parents

Before I close this chapter, I would like to include some questions from parents of children aged five to twelve, to draw together some of the information covered here. I hope you find them useful.

Q. *My five-year-old daughter is a very picky eater and I really struggle to get her to try anything new. She will not eat any* *fruit (not even in smoothies or juice) and the only vegetables she will touch are peas, raw carrot and sweetcorn, but she won't always eat them. She will eat pasta and cheese, potatoes and cheese and cheese sandwiches, but only white bread and definitely not butter. She will sometimes eat peanut butter on toast.*

I was parenting alone and was very anxious when I was weaning her onto solid foods, so didn't just let her play with food and enjoy the process of learning to eat. I was trying to do baby-led weaning but was really stressed about it, so I think she picked up on that. How can I encourage her to try new things? She freaks out if there's anything she doesn't like even near her.

A. I think you've hit the nail on the head when you say you feel that you didn't allow your daughter to enjoy the process of learning to eat when she was weaning onto solids. This is likely to have contributed to some of the issues she has with eating now. But the good news is that it is never too late to help her learn.

I think you must go back to basics and introduce the sensory side of eating that she missed out on as a baby, as well as including some steps to help familiarise her with food and feel more in control over her eating.

My suggestion would be to remove any pressure from the eating process. Initially, you need to accept your daughter and her eating. I would make sure that you offer a 'safe food' at each meal, so there is always something that she likes on her plate. Alongside this, I would introduce a new food or one that she has previously refused, but don't place any pressure on her to try it. If she voices her disdain, then just say, 'It's OK, you don't have to eat it if you don't want to'; and if she does try it, be sure to not praise her for doing so. You need to keep your responses to her eating neutral, whether you are happy or stressed with her.

To help her learn about food and, importantly, familiarise herself with it, I would consider setting up a fruit and vegetable garden with her. If you have a garden, think about creating a vegetable patch; if not, you can use just a couple of pots on a windowsill or balcony. Visit a garden centre together to look at seeds and ask her to choose what you're going to grow. Once home, encourage her to sow the seeds and take care of the plants as they grow. I would also try to take her food shopping with you as often as possible and ask her to get involved in your weekly meal planning, choosing dinners and lunches that you can both eat. She should be involved in meal preparation as much as possible, whether you are using ingredients you bought when shopping together, or harvested from your own plants. Encourage her to chop up the ingredients and handle them as much as possible. Try to really get her involved in the cooking process. You could look at cookery books together, selecting recipes you would like to try, making sure the books have photographs of the food and, even better, photographs of the raw ingredients. All this will help her to get to know different foods, which has been shown to slowly increase the variety of foods accepted and eaten.

I would also think about the example that you are setting her. How and what *you* eat has a tremendous influence on your daughter, so I would focus on eating a wide variety of foods yourself and limiting any picky eating behaviour you may have.

Finally, try to eat as many meals as possible with your daughter, and to make eating an enjoyable and relaxed experience that you share.

Q. *My seven-year-old has massive issues with body image. She cries that she is fat, wobbling her legs, and refuses to wear clothes that she thinks she looks fat in, even though* *she is slim. She has always had issues eating and has previously been seen by child mental-health professionals, who haven't helped. I am looking for any advice you have as to how to deal with this. I'm so scared this is going to be an eating disorder.*

A. Your daughter is not alone. A large percentage of girls, some as young as six years old, worry about their weight, especially believing that they are too fat.

First, I'm glad you have sought professional medical advice, and I would recommend that you ask for another appointment, perhaps with a different team if you don't have faith in the people you've already seen.

There are things you can do to help your daughter yourself, though, in the meantime. Your goal is to try to improve your daughter's body image and self-confidence and the most important place to start here is with yourself. You must be very careful that she is not picking up on any insecurities that you may have. Ban all talk of dieting in your house. You must try very hard to always speak positively about your own body and never say anything negative about the way you look in her presence. Similarly, avoid talking about other people's bodies, positively or negatively. Make sure that you never comment on your daughter's appearance – this includes praising her for her looks in any way. Instead, focus on paying her compliments for what she does, the actions she takes, what she says and things she achieves.

Next, you must be very careful about outside influences on your daughter. Keep a close eye on her Internet activity, including any videos she may watch online, and make sure that you filter any television she is exposed to, to exclude any programmes or adverts which focus on 'looking good', sexualising girls or showing them achieving anything – including happiness – based on their looks. Be careful about magazines or books that she reads too. I don't recommend any magazines specifically aimed at girls, as these all tend to focus heavily on appearance and being 'pretty'. With books, try to choose some that have a strong heroine who is popular and happy for being kind, brave, sporty or funny and remove any that focus on the characters being attractive. (Check out www.amightygirl.com for inspiration.) You should also be careful about the toys your daughter plays with, especially dolls that have very unrealistic, skinny bodies. You can get dolls that are more realistic and childlike.

I would also suggest that you try to encourage your daughter to find a hobby she enjoys and which allows her to meet regularly with like-minded peers. In addition, I would encourage her to find a sporting activity that she likes – perhaps cycling, climbing, tennis, swimming or a team sport. Make sure that you do not place any emphasis on the sport helping to keep her slim. Instead, focus on the fact that it's fun and will help her body to be strong.

When it comes to your daughter's eating, it should always be under her control, free of pressure from you to eat more or to eat more healthily. Again, don't praise her for eating 'well' or reward her for clearing her plate, as this is likely to backfire, causing her to have more anxiety about eating.

Q. *My son is eleven. We recently received a letter from his school, informing us that his BMI indicates that he is in the overweight range and he is at risk of becoming obese later in life. We genuinely have never had any worries about his weight. He is healthy, loves sport and plays in a local football team every weekend. He is tall for his age, but his weight is in proportion to his height. If anything, he is all muscle – there is no fat on him. Despite this, the letter has made us worried. Are we causing him problems? Is he perhaps overweight and we have missed it? Should we put him on a diet?*

A. I wouldn't put your son on a diet, for two reasons. First, he may not actually have a weight problem and second, diets really don't work.

BMI is not a reliable way to assess weight problems. As you say, your son is in proportion, weight and height, and an active boy, full of muscle. There is a strong chance that he doesn't actually have a weight problem. A more reliable way to assess potential weight issues is to look at the child's waist circumference in relation to their height. This gives a good idea of the amount of fat carried and where it is, which is a much more useful measurement than BMI. If you search 'waist-to-height ratio' on the Internet, you will find some example calculations and explanations of results. Sadly, this is not a measurement that schools are using at the moment.

That said, it is fairly common for parents to miss their own child's weight issues – that is, we tend to think they don't have a problem when they actually do. Even if your son is overweight, though, I would still not recommend that he diets. Restricting food only serves to make children think about it more and, ultimately, eat more. I would also avoid talking to your son about needing to lose weight, as this could cause him to seek food to palliate his emotions, or put himself on a diet, which will have the same pitfalls as if you were to put him on one. Instead, I would focus on helping your son to self-regulate his eating by making sure that there are no distractions at mealtimes that could make him overeat, such as eating while watching television or playing on a phone or tablet. Also, try to trust your son if he says he is full or hungry – don't encourage him to clear his plate – and don't question him if he says he is hungry, or restrict snacks.

Finally, it sounds as if your son is already active, with his football at the weekends. I would look at ways to increase his activity during the week, though, especially when he has been sitting down at school all day. An easy way to do this is to encourage him to walk or cycle to and from school each day, or find a sports club that trains on weekdays too.

The early school years may bring a whole host of new issues concerning childhood eating. However, if you understand their potential impact and work to follow gentle-eating principles, there is no reason why they cannot be navigated in a positive way to help children develop a healthy attitude to both eating and their bodies. The work you do at this stage will help you reap the rewards when your child enters their teenage years, when issues tend to be a continuation of those first experienced at a younger age, rather than any that are completely new. The next chapter focuses on exactly this.

Chapter 7

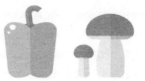

Teen Eating – Thirteen to Eighteen Years

What are the top eating issues that come to mind when you think about teenagers? The chances are that two of them will involve dieting and junk-food addiction – the picky eating of the teen years. It is simply not possible to write a chapter about teen eating without including these. I think it is also important to look at peer pressure and its effect on eating. And given the information in Chapter 1 on sleep and its impact on eating, we cannot ignore the effect of sleep on teenagers, who are known for their late nights and even later mornings, as well as the effect of screen use on sleep and, by extension, on eating.

At the end of this chapter I will focus on taking gentle-eating principles into adulthood. We need to consider how to prepare teens for living, and thus eating, independently – something that many are ill equipped for in today's society.

Let's start with the most pressing issues, though: dieting and junk food.

The dangerous world of teen dieting

Dieting becomes increasingly common in the teenage years, especially among girls, who are a lot more likely to want to lose weight than boys.[1] Family, friends and the media remain the biggest influences on dieting behaviour in teens.[2] The strength and type of close family relationships (such as sibling and parental) have an exceptionally powerful effect on teenage girls, with research showing that talk of weight, particularly by mothers, is linked with disordered eating:[3] 45 per cent of teenage girls questioned by researchers reported that their mothers had encouraged them to diet, while those girls whose mothers dieted displayed more extreme weight-control behaviour than those whose mothers did not.

It's not easy growing up in a world where you are bombarded with images of thinness; where 'plus size' is considered to be anything from a size fourteen up (US size ten), where fashion models promote size zero and magazines feature heavily photo-shopped images. Our children must contend with the selfie trend – something that we never had ourselves. And social media has undoubtedly played a central role in the rising trend of the healthy-living celebrity, with no social network as full of 'eating inspiration', or the commonly termed 'thinspiration', as Instagram. With 90 per cent of Instagram users aged under thirty-five, it is arguably the 'youngest' of all social-media networks. And research has shown that Instagram has a dark side when it comes to eating motivation, with 49 per cent of users questioned, who follow healthy living and eating-based accounts, displaying symptoms of orthorexia, in stark contrast to the 1 per cent incidence of the condition in the general pop-ulation.[4] This finding should be a wake-up call to the less than positive influence of social-media celebrities in the 'healthy-living' genre over hundreds of thousands of vulnerable teenage girls. In short, social media, celebrities and the impact of maternal dieting can cause teenage girls to pursue the thin ideal, resulting in body dissatisfaction, dieting and unhealthy weight control. Each of these behaviours increases the risk of bingeing, purging and other eating disorders.[5]

So how do we protect our daughters from the dangers of dieting? Once again, we must begin with ourselves. We must understand our own eating behaviour and we must stop dieting. If we, as parents, diet, we provide our teens with unnatural and unhealthy role models. We need to embrace our bodies, learn to eat more instinctively and speak positively about ourselves and others. Above all, we must resist the temptation to comment on the bodies of our children, whether they are over, under or the ideal weight.

Next, we cannot ignore the effects of social media. Minimum age requirements should be adhered to – they are there for a reason. My own children are only allowed social-media accounts if they add me as a friend and allow me to see everything they post and everybody they follow. I regularly monitor their activity and if I see anything that alarms me, we discuss it. I believe monitoring is even more important for teen girls on social media, particularly if they involve themselves in the 'healthy-living' community.

Moving for fun still applies in the teen years. Finding a sport or activity that your child enjoys can help to improve their confidence and body acceptance.

Finally, we must work hard to form close and meaningful relationships with our teens. Research has found that teenagers who have good-quality, positive relationships with their parents show better weight-related behaviours and fewer eating disorders.[6] Parents who fall into the authoritative parenting style that is part of gentle eating are far more likely to have a close and positive relationship with their children than those who follow the detached, strict, authoritarian parenting that is more in line with popular mainstream advice. Simply put, authoritative parenting protects teenagers from disordered eating.

It is a sobering – and scary – thought that, even in the teenage years, we still hold the most power over our children's behaviour. On the flip side, however, this realisation is cause for optimism because it means we can always do something to change things.

Junk-food addicts

At the opposite end of the disordered-eating spectrum to dieting lies the teenage version of picky eating – that of junk-food addiction. Where dieting affects significantly more girls than boys, junk-food addiction is more common in boys. Research has shown that 97 per cent of teenage boys consume 'fast food' occasionally and 14 per cent consume it every day.[7]

What causes this junk-food addiction? The answer is likely a blend of several factors. First, we must consider our own influence as parents. If we regularly eat junk food, then we are teaching our children to do the same. Proximity and availability obviously have an impact too, with research showing that teens are more likely to buy junk food if they pass an outlet to, or on the way home from, school.[8] Advertising and marketing have a big influence on eating behaviour and our teens are exposed to more of these today than ever before. Research has shown that television marketing of fast food not only improves recognition of the brand, but also influences teen eating behaviour, increasing the disposition towards eating junk food.[9] Social media plays a significant role too, with many sites showing advertising for junk-food brands targeted at teens and young adults, resulting in increased levels of engagement with the brands from this age bracket.[10] Finally, there is a distinct link between a teen's ability to regulate their emotions and emotional eating, specifically of junk food.[11] If teens are struggling with difficult emotions and are unable to find a healthy way to channel them, they are more likely to try to 'bury' them in eating and, when they do, they make poor food choices.

How do we try to gently steer teens away from junk-food addiction? Again, it requires a multi-factorial approach. There is no denying that picky eating from earlier in life can have an effect, so the advice already covered in this book for dealing with that still applies (see page 119). In addition, for teens, we need to spend time speaking to them about the power of advertising and helping them to spot common techniques used by marketers, thus enabling them to make informed choices about the food that they eat. Once again, we must also consider our relationship with our teens – knowing that emotional eating is more likely to involve junk food, we must help them to develop healthy alternative ways to cope with stress, anxiety and other uncomfortable emotions. Being open to conversation, whatever the subject, is important when helping teens to feel able to communicate their concerns to us, as their parents. Introducing them to techniques that can help them to regulate their emotions – such as yoga, mindfulness and meditation – can also be a good plan; and sporting activities can be helpful too. Once again, we also need to look at our own consumption of junk food, remembering that we model eating behaviour to our children.

There is one question that is not asked very often concerning teen junk-food consumption, but which, to me, seems the most obvious of all: do so many teens fill up on junk food because they are unable to prepare quick and healthy food themselves, perhaps because nobody has taught them? When you consider that it is mostly boys who fill up on junk food, this idea seems even more pertinent.

Preparing for independent living

The teenage years are a bridge between the full dependency of early childhood and the independence that is soon to be found in young adulthood. Many teens, however, are unprepared for independent living. I remember starting university, living away from home for the first time at eighteen, and noticing how many of my peers were unable to cook even the simplest of meals. The boys seemed to live on a diet of instant noodles, bacon sandwiches and McDonald's, simply because of their inability to prepare healthier foods.

I firmly believe that by the end of their teen years, all children or young adults as they are then, should be competent not only at cooking, but also meal planning, grocery shopping and budgeting. Sadly, these subjects are inadequately covered at school. Cookery lessons are scant at best and not a core part of the national curriculum past the age of fourteen. Meal planning and budgeting are not covered at all. So if parents do not teach their children these basic life skills, is it any wonder teens are unable to take care of themselves in a healthy way?

We must take time to teach our teens or, preferably, younger children about meal planning, budgeting, grocery shopping and cooking at home because we cannot rely on their formal education to cover these areas.

The pressures of fitting in

Pressure from peers and the desire to fit in are another challenge presented in the teenage years, as children become increasingly independent and spend more time eating away from home.

Research shows that eating with peers massively distorts how much teenagers eat, with girls eating 33 per cent less food than normal and boys eating 23 per cent more.[12] Teens also eat considerably more unhealthy food in the presence of peers who are doing so – unsurprisingly, the effects here are stronger for boys than girls. Best friends, in particular, tend to have a matched daily energy intake, exerting the most influence of all.[13] To counteract some of this behaviour, we must empower our teens to embrace their individuality. Indeed, empowerment is one of the tenets of gentle eating.

So how do you help teens to feel empowered? It starts earlier in life, when you respect their eating behaviour, trust them to respond to their bodily cues and accept their likes and dislikes. Your relationship with your teen can, once again, help them to feel confident in themselves and to know their own mind and own body, which can, in turn, allow them to resist the peer pressure around eating.

Avoiding teen eating pitfalls

Teens are famed for their quick tempers, sulks, exam stress, burning the midnight oil and poor sleep habits. Chapter 1 looked at the impact of stress and sleep on our eating, and if we want our teens to develop the healthiest possible relationship with food, we must consider the way they cope with this.

Stress

The teenage years are undeniably a stressful period. From puberty and friendship issues, school work, homework, exams and university applications, to clashes with parents – teens have to cope with a level of stress beyond any they have ever dealt with before. So the role of parents here is important. In order to prevent emotional eating, or eating as a way to handle pressure, we need to try to remove as much of it as possible and provide our teens with healthy and proactive ways to cope.

Discussing stress and its impact on our bodies is important, as is having a conversation about healthy and unhealthy ways to cope with it. It is a sad reality that teens today need stress-management techniques. Even if we manage to remove as much stress as possible from their home life, they still need to cope with school-related pressure, which appears to be on the increase with the ever-changing demands placed on teens to score higher in exams.

Giving teens some tools with which to manage their emotions empowers them in such a way that they are better equipped to follow gentle-eating principles. Here are some techniques that can work especially well:

- Listening to a mindfulness or relaxation app, downloaded onto their phone or tablet.

- Practising gratitude and altruistic behaviour. Volunteering for charity work can give teenagers a real sense of purpose and can help them to appreciate what they have, when helping others less fortunate.

- Finding a new hobby or a new sporting activity, particularly if they feel included as part of a team, or group of like-minded individuals.

- Attending a teen yoga or Pilates class – encouraging them to feel more 'at one' with their bodies, while also taking time out to unwind and relax.

- Attending a teen activity holiday scheme or retreat; the increase in popularity of 'teenager retreats' is surely testament to the rising levels of stress that so many experience today.

Sleep

We know that late nights and insufficient sleep play havoc with ghrelin and leptin levels (see page 12), ultimately resulting in weight gain. A lack of sleep also affects our immune system, causing more frequent colds and other viruses, and impacts on our cognitive function and academic performance. Research shows that teens today get an average of seven hours sleep per night, although recommendations are that they get somewhere between eight and ten.[14] This sleep deficit poses a real danger to teens, their weight and their overall health and wellbeing. Parents need to address this with their teens, helping them to avoid the common pitfalls that have a negative impact on sleep. Here are some of the important points to consider regarding sleep hygiene:

- Research has shown that teens who keep to a parentally set and enforced bedtime have more sleep and less weight gain than those who do not.[15]

- Avoid exposure to screens (televisions, phones, tablets and computers) for at least one hour before bed. The light from these devices is known to inhibit the secretion of melatonin, the sleep hormone, thus interfering with the onset of sleep.

- Restrict video-game playing, especially in the evening.[16] The light emitted from the screens poses an issue, but, in addition, the stimulation from the games makes it harder for the brain to switch off and rest.

- Restrict caffeinated drinks, especially in the run-up to bed-time.

- Keep bedrooms as dark and cool as possible in order to not inhibit the secretion of melatonin, which decreases in the presence of heat as well as light.

- Follow a good winding-down and bedtime routine each evening.

Helping teens to keep themselves healthy, and empowering them to take more control over their lives in preparation for the increase in independence they will shortly face, is perhaps the greatest gift parents can give to their child. Keeping the doors of communication open, giving non-judgemental advice when it is asked for, and providing a reliable base to return to when they are in need are also important.

Healthy eating in the teen years requires parents to adopt a holistic approach, which can be summed up by the principles of gentle eating. Let's remind ourselves of the main tenets once more. Gentle eating is:

- mindful

- empowering

- respectful

- authoritative.

Gentle eating throughout the teen years focuses very much on shifting the balance of power even more towards the child, in preparation for independent living and adulthood. As ever, parents should be mindful of their actions, and how their beliefs impact on their teens, in order to empower them to maintain a good relationship with food and their own bodies. Affording teens control over their eating as much as possible, through an authoritative parenting style, helps them to feel respected; this, in turn, is likely to lead to a good level of self-respect and self-esteem, both of which are a key influence on eating patterns.

Questions from parents

Let's close this chapter with questions from two parents, concerning their teens' eating behaviour. As you read through them, and my responses, think back to the topics we have discussed and how the information can be applied to real-life situations.

Q. *My fourteen-year-old son has been a picky eater for as long as I can remember. As a younger child, he would eat a monotonous diet, although it did include most food groups. I tried not to let it bother me, but goaded by well-meaning advice from relatives, I made every mealtime a battle with threats, bribes, hidden food or lies about ingredients. Over time, I realised this wasn't working and relaxed, including allowing him to eat whatever he wanted from a meal with no comments about 99 per cent of the time.*

However, he now has an intense mistrust of food, alongside an even more restricted diet. He goes the whole day at school with only an apple and packet of crisps, then comes home and makes a chocolate-spread wrap or hot dog. He generally eats very little of any dinner I make, unless it's one of three trusted meals. He doesn't get ill often, and probably just about gets by with most nutrients right now, but I'm concerned about his long-term health. Is there a way to improve his trust and relationship with food? Will this issue extend into adulthood?

A. There is a fair amount of information and support for picky eating in early childhood, however nobody really seems to talk about picky eating in the teen years, even though it is still common, especially among boys.

You have already discovered that bribery, reward and punishment are not the way forward. Relinquishing control over what and how your son eats is definitely the best approach. I would, however, pay a little more attention to what you are offering him. You mention that he has three trusted meals. This is a good start. Each day I would offer dinner that includes at least one trusted and accepted food. Alongside this, I would serve a challenging food, whether that is a new or previously discarded one, and would pay attention to the iron levels in the food offered. I would put no pressure on your son to eat, or even try the food though. I would discuss nutritional needs with your son, but you must approach this in a very non-judgemental and non-confrontational way. Help him to understand what his body needs to grow and stay healthy and what happens if he is lacking in certain nutrients, but make sure you do not put any pressure on him to change his eating.

It may be that your son would benefit from a vitamin and mineral supplement in the interim, although you should make it clear to him that supplements are not a replacement for eating and, as such, they are not a quick fix.

Involve your son in food as much as possible at home. Encourage him to help plan your meals and, most importantly, to help make them. Including him in food preparation and cooking as much as possible will not only help him to feel more at ease with food, but will also get him ready for the coming years when you will no longer be on hand to make his meals for him. I would experiment with different styles of cooking – for instance, food cooked on a barbecue may suit him more than that cooked indoors with a conventional oven. I would also try different cuisines; he may find making sushi more fun than traditional Western cookery, for example.

It is important that you think about the eating behaviours you are modelling too. Are you as adventurous about eating as you could be? Do you tend to snack on fast food? What can you improve about your own eating habits?

I would also work hard on your relationship with your son.

We know that teens who have a slightly difficult relationship with their parents can tend to eat more junk food. Are there any cracks in your relationship that need to be fixed? Are you as supportive as you could be? Think about ways in which you can make your relationship stronger, perhaps by planning a special day out or picking up a new hobby that you can both enjoy together.

Above all, though, you must accept your son unconditionally, eating habits and all. The more your son feels accepted by you and the less he feels you are trying to change him, the better his eating is likely to be.

Q. *My daughter is fourteen and has recently become obsessed with her weight. She has never been a skinny child, but she is definitely not fat. Her two closest friends are quite skinny and she keeps saying that she feels fat in comparison to them. I have tried to talk to her about everybody being different, but it doesn't seem to have helped. She is getting very picky about what she eats and is deliberately avoiding certain foods if they have more than a little fat or sugar in them. I am worried about where this may lead. Do you have any advice?*

A. Dieting and concerns about weight are unfortunately common in the teen years, especially with girls. I think you need to start with thinking about where your daughter's beliefs may stem from. We know that teens pick up on messages about weight and body shape from their friends and the media. I would be concerned about any potential weight-related teasing at school – teenage girls can be really quite mean to each other. I would also want to keep an eye on the magazines and books she reads and what she watches, especially online videos. An extremely worrying source of media 'thinspiration' is social media. If your daughter has social-media accounts, particularly Instagram, I would want to know exactly what information she was picking up on and who is influencing her. Social-media 'healthy-living' celebrities can often spread quite worrying information concerning eating, especially when their audience is vulnerable teenage girls.

Perhaps the biggest influence on teen body image, however, is you. Your own eating behaviour and body image will have a direct effect on your daughter. Think about the relationship you have with your own body and what your self-talk says about your beliefs. Are you constantly complaining about needing to lose weight? Or do you show gratitude and acceptance of the body that you have. If you diet at all, you will have an impact on your daughter and not in a good way. Coming to terms with your own body is possibly the most important thing you can do to set a good example to your daughter. Also, be careful to not comment on her body in *any* way – even the most well-intentioned and positive comments can spark negative feelings in her about her body.

Finally, you really need to increase your daughter's confidence and feelings of acceptance. Your relationship with her is key. Perhaps it's time for some mother–daughter bonding away from the stresses and distractions of everyday life? I would also recommend that you help your daughter to find a hobby that she loves – better still if it is one related to sport, so she can begin to value her body for all that it can do, rather than what it looks like. It would be great if you could be involved in this new activity with her too.

Summary

I want to close this book with a summary of the fundamental points covered. To do this, it makes sense to revisit the ethos of gentle eating and to reiterate the four key elements. Gentle eating is all of the following:

1. Mindful

Gentle eating is informed. That means being aware of the different physiological processes involved in hunger and satiation and the various elements that can inhibit our body's natural cycles (covered in Chapter 1). There are many ways in which we commonly derail instinctive eating and turn it into something governed by emotions, inherited beliefs and messages given to us by society. Gentle eating means breaking free of these unhealthy beliefs and returning to a mindful and conscious way of eating. It means removing distractions and emotions, and not projecting our worries onto our children or repeating unhealthy inherited patterns of eating.

2. Empowering

Gentle eating focuses on responsive feeding, encouraging children to develop self-regulation skills as early as possible in their lives. Empowering means giving children control – over what they eat, when they eat, how they eat and how much they eat. It means no bribing or rewarding them to eat, no banning or restricting foods, no calorie counting or following diets that don't work. Gentle eating means setting our children free of *our* eating hang-ups and giving them the freedom to enjoy eating.

3. Respectful

Gentle eating means respecting our children's hunger and satiation levels. It means learning to trust that they know what is best for their own bodies. To show children respect we need to honour their likes and dislikes and understand and accept that their food preferences may not be the same as ours.

4. Authoritative

Gentle eating means having an authoritative parenting style, not an authoritarian one. It means allowing our children to have as much autonomy over their eating as possible. Gentle eating is child-led and child-friendly. Children are at the heart of the approach and at the centre of their eating. Gentle, authoritative eating means working at the pace and developmental stage of the child, not expecting eating-related behaviour from them that is unrealistic for their age.

*

As I hope is now apparent, the principles of gentle eating apply at any age, from the day your baby is born to the day your teenager leaves home. At its heart, always, are respect and understanding.

Gentle eating is an ethos, or a lifestyle change, rather than a quick-fix, one-size-fits-all solution. It means re-educating ourselves and stripping away the paranoia, worries and concerns that stem from our own upbringing. It means looking at eating afresh, through newly informed eyes.

The principles of gentle eating are preparation for life and the results are lifelong. While you may not see any of those results for several months, or even years, when you do see them they will be the healthiest, most long-lasting and the gentlest possible for your child. Some come to gentle eating at the very beginning of their children's lives, some discover it several years down the line, after realising that common, mainstream ways of tackling eating problems are not only ineffective, but potentially more damaging than the problems they seek to resolve. The beauty of gentle eating is that it is never too late to make a change.

Gentle eating usually requires that we change just as much, if not more, than our children. Most of our children's eating issues belong to us, or stem from our beliefs and behaviours. Many go back generations. Very often, learning about your child's eating can uncover all sorts of issues with your own eating habits that you didn't know existed. This knowledge can sometimes be painful. Therefore, gentle eating requires that you are gentle with yourself too. To make the changes that are necessary to break the eating cycles of your own family and to do what is best for your children, you need to embrace a degree of introspection – forgiving yourself for any lack of awareness of the roots of your approach to eating.

When you are the parent of a picky, underweight or overweight child you can feel inadequate, guilty, shamed and more. All too often, parents are criticised for the way they feed their children, and this criticism, doubt and guilt can cause fractures in the parent–child relationship. Gentle eating requires parents to have enough confidence to trust in their children and the ethos of gentle eating. This can often be tricky, considering the conflicting messages received from society. Here, gentleness towards yourself is once again vital. To help your child, you must have the courage to break free of the current beliefs that may have been restraining you.

Eating should be an enjoyable process, not something that is accompanied by stress and anxiety. One of the best ways to stay on track is to build your confidence at the same time as building your child's. Shared activities can help to take the stress out of everyday life and the time spent together is a much-needed bonding exercise that can go some way to removing the wedge that picky or overeating may have driven between you and your child. Together, with trust and with confidence, you can take the brave steps necessary to embrace gentle eating.

I hope that this book has given you the assurance and inspiration you need to not only help your child to develop psychologically and physiologically positive, healthy eating habits, but to make a change in your own for the better too.

Gentle eating is a blueprint for normal and healthy eating at any age or stage of life, whatever eating issue you may be facing. I hope that it changes your life as much as it has mine. There is no greater feeling than breaking free of the hold that food has over your family and finally learning to embrace the joy of eating.

Useful Resources

Babies

Kelly Mom breastfeeding information site www.kellymom.com
La Leche League breastfeeding support www.llli.org
Reflux information and support www.livingwithreflux.org
Tongue tie information and support www.tonguetie.net
International Association of Lactation Consultants
      www.ilca.org

Eating disorders

Anorexia and bulimia support www.b-eat.co.uk
Orthorexia information site www.orthorexia.com
Young Minds, for the wellbeing of young people
      www.youngminds.org.uk

Food allergies and food-related diseases

Allergy UK support and information www.allergyuk.org
Coeliac UK support and information www.coeliac.org.uk

Gentle eating for adults

Beyond Chocolate, the no-dieting community
    www.beyondchocolate.co.uk
Intuitive eating information www.intuitiveeating.com

Girls and positive body image

Body Gossip www.bodygossip.co.uk
Just Between Us journal www.chroniclebooks.com
A Mighty Girl – book and toy suggestions
    www.amightygirl.com

Special-eating needs

Sensory processing disorder, Star Institute www.spdstar.com
Tube feeding www.feedingtubeawareness.org

Resources on social media

The Gentle Eating Book on Facebook
    www.facebook.com/The-Gentle-Eating-Book
Sarah Ockwell-Smith on Facebook
    www.facebook.com/sarahockwellsmithauthor
Sarah Ockwell-Smith on Twitter
    www.twitter.com/TheBaby Expert
Sarah Ockwell-Smith on Instagram
    www.instagram.com/sarahockwellsmith
Sarah Ockwell-Smith's Blog
    www.sarahockwell-smith.com

References

Chapter 1

1. Plata-Salaman, C., 'Regulation of hunger and satiety in man', *Digestive Diseases*, 9 (5) (1991): pp. 253–68.
2. Amin, T. and Mercer, J., 'Hunger and satiety mechanisms and their potential exploitation in the regulation of food intake', *Current Obesity Reports*, 5 (2016): pp. 106–12.
3. Havermans, R., Janssen, T., Giesen, J. and Roefs, A., 'Food liking, food wanting, and sensory-specific satiety', *Appetite*, 52 (1) (2009): pp. 222–5.
4. Taheri, S., Lin, S., Austin, D., Young, T. and Mignot, E., 'Short sleep duration is associated with reduced leptin, elevated ghrelin, and increased body mass index', *PLoS Medicine*, 1 (3) (2004), e62.
5. Prinz, P., 'Sleep, appetite, and obesity – what is the link?', *PLoS Medicine*, 1 (3) (2004), e61.
6. Lutter, M., Sakata, I., Osborne-Lawrence, S., Rovinsky, S., Anderson, J., Jung, S., Birnbaum, S., Yanagisawa, M., Elmquist, J., Nestler, E. and Zigman, J., 'The orexigenic hormone ghrelin defends against depressive symptoms of chronic stress', *Nature Neuroscience*, 11 (7) (2008): pp. 752–3.
7. Epel, E., Lapidus, R., McEwen, B. and Brownell, K., 'Stress may add bite to appetite in women: a laboratory study of stress-induced cortisol and eating behavior', *Psychoneuroendocrinology*, 26 (1) (2001): pp. 37–49.
8. Yau, Y. and Potenza, M., 'Stress and eating behaviors', *Minerva Endocrinology*, 38 (3) (2013): pp. 255–67.

Chapter 2

1. Vollmer, R. and Baietto, J., 'Practices and preferences: exploring the relationships between food-related parenting practices and child food preferences for high fat and/or sugar foods, fruits, and vegetables', *Appetite* (1 June 2017), pp. 134–40.
2. Powell, E., Frankel, L. and Hernandez, D., 'The mediating role of child self-regulation of eating in the relationship between parental use of food as a reward and child emotional overeating', *Appetite* (1 June 2017), pp. 78–83.
3. Koenigstorfer, J., 'The effect of fitness branding on restrained eaters' food consumption and postconsumption physical activity', *Journal of Marketing Research*, 53 (1) (2016): pp. 124–38.
4. Maimaran, M. and Fishbach, A., 'If it's useful and you know it, do you eat? Preschoolers refrain from instrumental food', *Journal of Consumer Research*, 41 (3) (2014): pp. 642–55.
5. Crum, A., Corbin, W., Brownell, K. and Salovey, P., 'Mind over milkshake: mindsets, not just nutrients, determine ghrelin response', *Health Psychology*, 30 (4) (2011): pp. 424–9.
6. Tatangelo, G., McCabe, M., Mellor, D. and Mealey, A., 'A systematic review of body dissatisfaction and sociocultural messages related to the body among preschool children', *Body Image*, 18 (2016): pp. 86–95; Garbett, K. and Diedrichs, P., 'Improving uptake and engagement with child body image interventions delivered to mothers: understanding mother and daughter preferences for intervention content', *Body Image*, 19 (2016): pp. 24–7.
7. 'Attitudes towards Healthy Eating – UK', February 2016, Mintel Market Intelligence Report.
8. Mann, T., Tomiyama, A., Westling, E., Lew, A., Samuels, B. and Chatman, J., 'Medicare's search for effective obesity treatments: diets are not the answer', *American Psychologist*, 62 (3) (2007): pp. 220–33.
9. Pietiläinen, K., 'Does dieting make you fat? A twin study', *International Journal of Obesity*, 36 (3) (2012): pp. 456–64.
10. Field, A., 'Relation between dieting and weight change among preadolescents and adolescents', *Pediatrics*, 112 (2003): pp. 900–6.
11. Coffman, D., Balantekin, K. and Savage, J., 'Using propensity score methods to assess causal effects of mothers' dieting behavior on daughters' early dieting behavior', *Childhood Obesity*, 12 (5) (2016): pp. 334–40.

12. The Bratman Orthorexia Test, accessed online, 6 March 2017: http://www.orthorexia.com/the-authorized-bratman-orthorexia-self-test/.

Chapter 3

1. Cunnington, A., Sim, K., Deierl, A., Kroll, J., Brannigan E. and Darby, J., '"Vaginal seeding" of infants born by Caesarean section', *BMJ*, 352 (2016).
2. Cruchet, S., et al., 'The use of probiotics in pediatric gastroenterology: a review of the literature and recommendations by Latin-American experts', *Pediatric Drugs* (2015), 17(3): 199–216; Wang, Q., Dong, J. and Zhu, Y., 'Probiotic supplement reduces risk of necrotizing enterocolitis and mortality in preterm very low-birth-weight infants: an updated meta-analysis of 20 randomized, controlled trials', *Journal of Pediatric Surgery* (January 2012), 47(1): 241–8.
3. Mansfield, J., Bergin, S., Cooper, J. and Olsen, C., 'Comparative probiotic strain efficacy in the prevention of eczema in infants and children: a systematic review and meta-analysis', *Military Medicine* (Jun 2014), 179(6): 580–92.
4. Kent, G., 'The high price of infant formula in the United States', Department of Political Science, University of Hawaii, accessed online, 8 March 2017: http://www2.hawaii.edu/~kent/The%20High%20Price%20of%20Infant%20Formula%20in%20the%20US.pdf.
5. Ingram, J., 'Multiprofessional training for breastfeeding management in primary care in the UK', *International Breastfeeding Journal* (April 2006), 1: 9.
6. 'Global strategy for infant and young child feeding', World Health Organization, accessed online, 8 March 2017: http://apps.who.int/iris/bitstream/10665/42590/1/9241562218.pdf.
7. Guidance Notes on the Infant Formula and Follow-on Formula regulations, accessed online, 8 March 2017: https://www.gov.uk/government/uploads/system/uploads/attachment_data/file/204314/Infant_formula_guidance_2013_-_final_6_March.pdf.
8. Iacovou, M. and Sevilla, A., 'Infant feeding: the effects of scheduled vs. on-demand feeding on mothers' wellbeing and children's cognitive development', *European Journal of Public Health* (February 2013), 23(1): 13–19.
9. Dinkevich, E., Leid, L., Pryor, K., Wei, Y., Huberman, H. and

Carnell, S., 'Mothers' feeding behaviors in infancy: do they predict child weight trajectories?' *Obesity* (2015), 23(12): 2470–6; Gross, R., Mendelsohn, A., Fierman, A., Hauser, N. and Messito, M., 'Maternal infant feeding behaviors and disparities in early child obesity', *Childhood Obesity* (2014), 10(2): 145–52.

10. World Health Organization. Infant and Young Child Feeding factsheet, September 2016. http://www.who.int/mediacentre/factsheets/fs342/en/.

11. Hohman, E., Paul, I. M., Birch, L. and Savage, J., 'INSIGHT responsive parenting intervention is associated with healthier patterns of dietary exposures in infants', *Obesity* (January 2017), 25(1): 185–91.

12. Hetherington, M., 'Understanding infant eating behaviour – lessons learned from observation', *Physiology and Behaviour*, (12 January 2017), epub ahead of print; Shloim, N., Vereiiken, C., Blundell, P., Hetherington, M., 'Looking for cues – infant communication of hunger and satiation during milk feeding', *Appetite* (1 January 2017), 108: 74–82.

13. 'Helping Your Baby to Sleep', NHS Choices, accessed online, 9 March 2017: http://www.nhs.uk/Conditions/pregnancy-and-baby/pages/getting-baby-to-sleep.aspx.

14. Ben-Joseph, E., Dowshen, S. and Izenberg, N., 'Do parents understand growth charts? A national, internet-based survey', *Pediatrics*, (2009), 124: 4.

15. Harlow, H., Dodsworth, R. and Harlow, M., 'Total social isolation in monkeys', *Proceedings of the National Academy of Sciences, USA*, 1965.

Chapter 4

1. Fildes, V., 'Infant feeding practices and infant mortality in England, 1900–1919', *Continuity and Change* (1998), 13(2): 251–80.

2. Department of Health, *Weaning and the Weaning Diet, Report of the Working Group on the Weaning Diet of the Committee on Medical Aspects of Food Policy (Reports on Health and Social Subjects)* (1994), 45, 1–113.

3. Hamlyn, B., Brooker, S., Oleinikova, K. and Wands, S., 'Infant Feeding 2000' (May 2002).

4. World Health Organization, 'Global strategy for infant and young child feeding. The optimal duration of exclusive breastfeeding', 54th World Health Assembly (2001).

5. European Food Safety Authority (EFSA) Panel, 'Dietetic products, nutrition and allergies (NDA), scientific opinion on the appropriate age for introduction of complementary feeding of infants', *EFSA Journal* (2009), 7(12): 1423–61.

6. NHMRC Dietary Guidelines for Children and Adolescents in Australia (1995); Dewey, K., Heinig, M., Nommsen, L. and Lonnerdal, B., 'Maternal versus infant factors related to breast milk intake and residual milk volume: the DARLING study', *Pediatrics* (June 1991), 87(6): 829–37; Food and Drug Administration (FDA), 'Food labeling: reference daily intakes, part II; final rule', *Federal Register* (1995), 60: 67, 164–67175.

7. Griffin, J. and Abrams, S., 'Iron and breastfeeding', *Pediatric Clinics of North America* (April 2001), 48(2): 401–13.

8. Kc, A., Rana, N., Malqvist, M., Jarawka, R., Subedi, K. and Andersson, O., 'Effects of delayed umbilical cord clamping vs early clamping on anemia in infants at 8 and 12 months: a randomized clinical trial', *JAMA Pediatrics* (1 March 2017), 171(3): 264–70.

9. McMillan, J., Oski, F., Lourie, G., Tomarelli, R. and Landaw, S., 'Iron absorption from human milk, simulated human milk, and proprietary formulas', *Pediatrics* (December 1977), 60(6): 896–900.

10. Zamzam, K., Zito, C. and Hunt, R., 'Initial uptake and absorption of nonheme iron and absorption of heme iron in humans are unaffected by the addition of calcium as cheese to a meal with high iron bioavailability', *American Journal of Clinical Nutrition* (August 2002), 76(2): 419–25.

11. 'Public Health England recommends vitamin D supplements in autumn and winter', *BMJ* (21 July 2016), 354.

12. 'Vitamins for Children', NHS Choices, accessed online, 13 March 2017: http://www.nhs.uk/Conditions/pregnancy-and-baby/pages/vitamins-for-children.aspx.

13. Wagner, C. and Greer, F., 'Prevention of rickets and vitamin D deficiency in infants, children, and adolescents', *Pediatrics* (November 2008), 122(4): 908–10.

14. Clayton, H., Li, R., Perrine, C. and Scanlon, K., 'Prevalence and reasons for introducing infants early to solid foods: variations by milk feeding type', *Pediatrics* (April 2013), 131(4): e1108–14.

15. Smith, H. and Becker, G., 'Early additional food and fluids for healthy breastfed full-term infants', *Cochrane Database Systematic Review* (30 Aug 2016) (8).

16. Keane, V., 'Do solids help baby sleep through the night?', *American Journal of Diseases of Childhood* (1988), 142: 404–05.

17. Brown, A. and Harries, V., 'Infant sleep and night feeding patterns during later infancy: association with breastfeeding frequency, daytime complementary food intake and infant weight', *Breastfeeding Medicine* (June 2015), 10(5): 246–52.

18. 'Your Baby's First Solid Foods', NHS Choices, accessed online, 13 March 2017: http://www.nhs.uk/Conditions/pregnancy-and-baby/Pages/solid-foods-weaning.aspx.

19. 'Weaning Your Baby Onto Solids', Allergy UK, accessed online, 13 March 2017: http://www.allergyuk.org/advice-for-parents-with-a-new-baby/weaning-your-baby-on-to-solids.

20. 'Feeding a New Baby', Coeliac UK, accessed online, 13 March 2017: https://www.coeliac.org.uk/gluten-free-diet-and-lifestyle/support-for-parents/babies/.

21. Brown, A. and Lee, M., 'A descriptive study investigating the use and nature of baby-led weaning in a UK sample of mothers', *Maternal and Child Nutrition* (January 2011), 7(1): 34–47.

22. Cameron, S., Taylor, R. and Heath, A., 'Parent-led or baby-led? Associations between complementary feeding practices and health-related behaviours in a survey of New Zealand families', *BMJ Open* (December 2013), 9: 3(12).

23. Brown, A. and Lee, M., 'Early influences on child satiety-responsiveness: the role of weaning style', *Pediatric Obesity* (February 2015), 10(1): 57–66.

24. Morison, B., Taylor, R., Hashard, J. and Schramm, C., 'How different are baby-led weaning and conventional complementary feeding? A cross-sectional study of infants aged 6–8 months', *BMJ Open* (May 2016), 6(5).

25. Cameron, S., Taylor, R. and Heath, A., 'Development and pilot testing of baby-led introduction to solids – a version of baby-led weaning modified to address concerns about iron deficiency, growth faltering and choking', *BMC Pediatrics* (2015), 26(15): 99.

26. Davis, M., 'Assessment of human dietary exposure to arsenic through rice', *The Science of the Total Environment*, 20 February 2017, epub ahead of print.

27. Mok, E., Vanstone, C., Gallo, S., Li, P., Constantin, E. and Weiler, H., 'Diet diversity, growth and adiposity in healthy breastfed infants fed homemade complementary foods', *International Journal of Obesity*, 7 March 2017, epub ahead of print.

28. Foterek, K., Hilbig, A. and Alexy, U., 'Associations between commercial complementary food consumption and fruit and vegetable intake in children. Results of the DONALD study',

Appetite (February 2015), 85: 84–90; Mennella, J. and Trabulsi, J., 'Complementary foods and flavor experiences: setting the foundation', *Annals of Nutrition and Metabolism* (2012), 60(2): 40–50.

29. Fangupo, L., Heath, A. and Williams, S., 'A baby-led approach to eating solids and risk of choking', *Pediatrics* (October 2016), 138(4).

30. Ventura, A. and Worobey, J., 'Early influences on the development of food preferences', *Current Biology* (6 May 2013), 23(9): R401–8.

31. Li, R., Magadia, J., Fein, S. and Grummer-Strawn, L., 'Risk of bottle-feeding for rapid weight gain during the first year of life', *Archives of Pediatric and Adolescent Medicine* (May 2012), 166(5): 431–6.

Chapter 5

1. Nicklaus, S., 'Development of food variety in children', *Appetite* (2009), 52(1), 253–5.

2. Mauch, C., Magarey, A., Byrne, R. and Daniels, L., 'Serve sizes and frequency of food consumption in Australian children aged 14 and 24 months', *Australia and New Zealand Journal of Public Health* (February 2017), 41(1): 38–44.

3. Reed, D. and Knaapila, A., 'Genetics of taste and smell: poisons and pleasures', *Progress of Molecular Biology and Translational Science Journal* (2010), 94: 213–40.

4. Mennella, J., Pepino, M., Duke, F. and Reed, D., 'Age modifies the genotype-phenotype relationship for the bitter receptor TAS2R38', *BMC Genetics* (2010), 11: 60.

5. Fildes, A., van Jaarsveld, C., Llewellyn, C., Fisher, A., Cooke, L. and Wardle, J., 'Nature and nurture in children's food preferences', *American Journal of Clinical Nutrition* (April 2014), 99(4): 911–7.

6. Fildes, A., van Jaarsveld, C., Cooke, L., Wardle, J., Fisher, A. and Llewellyn, C., 'Common genetic architecture underlying young children's food fussiness and liking for vegetables and fruit', *American Journal of Clinical Nutrition* (April 2016), 103(4): 1099–104.

7. Powell, F., Farrow, C. and Meyer, C., 'Food avoidance in children. The influence of maternal feeding practices and behaviours', *Appetite* (2011), 57(3): 683–92.

8. Wethmann, J., Jansen, A., Havermans, R., Nederkoom, C.,

Kreme, S. and Roefs, A., (2015), 'Bits and pieces. Food texture influences food acceptance in young children', *Appetite* (January 2015), 84: 181–7.

9.   Johnson, S., Davies, P., Boles, R., Gavin, W. and Bellows, L., 'Young children's food neophobia characteristics and sensory behaviors are related to their food intake', *Journal of Nutrition* (November 2015), 145(11): 2610–6.

10. Brown, C., Pesch, M., Perrin, E., Appugliese, D., Miller, A., Rosenblum, K. and Lumeng, J., 'Maternal concern for child undereating', *Academic Pediatrics* (November–December 2016), 16(8): 777–82.

11. Mosli, R., Lumend, J., Kaciroti, N., Peterson, K., Rosenblum, K., Baylin, A. and Miller, A., 'Higher weight status of only and last-born children. Maternal feeding and child eating behaviors as underlying processes among 4–8 year olds', *Appetite* (September 2015), 92: 167–72.

12. Cooke, L., Chambers, L., Anez, E. and Wardle, J., 'Facilitating or undermining? The effect of reward on food acceptance. A narrative review', *Appetite* (October 2011), 57(2): 493–7.

13. Fries, L., Martin, N. and van der Horst, K., 'Parent-child mealtime interactions associated with toddlers' refusals of novel and familiar foods', *Physiology and Behaviour*, 14 March 2017), epub ahead of print.

14. Gibson, E. and Cooke, L., 'Understanding food fussiness and its implications for food choice, health, weight and interventions in young children: the impact of professor Jane Wardle', *Current Obesity Reports* (16 February 2017), epub ahead of print.

15. Orrell-Valent, J., Hill, L., Brechwald, W., Dodge, K., Pettit, G. and Bates, J., '"Just three more bites": an observational analysis of parents' socialization of children's eating at mealtime', *Appetite*, 48 (1) (2007): pp. 37–45.

16. Birch, L. and Fisher, J., 'Development of eating behaviors among children and adolescents', *Pediatrics*, 101 (3 pt 2) (1998): pp. 539–49.

17. Coulthard, H. and Sealy, A., 'Play with your food! Sensory play is associated with tasting of fruits and vegetables in preschool children', *Appetite*, 113 (2017): 84–90.

18. Heath, P., Houston-Price, C. and Kennedy, O., 'Let's look at leeks! Picture books increase toddlers' willingness to look at, taste and consume unfamiliar vegetables', *Frontiers in Psychology* 5 (2014): p. 191.

19. Addessi, E., Galloway, A., Visalberghi, E. and Birch, L., 'Specific

social influences on the acceptance of novel foods in 2–5-year-old children', *Appetite*, 45 (3) (2005): pp. 264–71.

20. Edelson, L., Mokdad, C. and Martin, N., 'Prompts to eat novel and familiar fruits and vegetables in families with 1–3 year-old children: relationships with food acceptance and intake', *Appetite*, 1 (99) (2016): pp. 138–48.

21. De Barse, L., Cardona Cano, S., Jansen, P., Jaddoe, V., Verhulst, F., Franco, O., Tiemeir, H. and Tharner, A. (2016), 'Are parents' anxiety and depression related to child fussy eating?', *Archives of Diseases in Childhood*, 101 (6) (2016): pp. 533–8.

22. Perry, L., Samuelson, L. and Burdinie, J., 'Highchair philosophers: the impact of seating context-dependent exploration on children's naming biases', *Developmental Science*, 17 (5) (2014): pp. 757–65.

Chapter 6

1. Kakinami, L., Barnett, R., Sequin, L. and Paradis, G. 'Parenting style and obesity risk in children', *Preventive Medicine* (June 2015), 75: pp. 18–22.

2. Evans, C., Cleghorn, C., Greenwood, D. and Cade, J., 'A comparison of British school meals and packed lunches from 1990 to 2007: meta-analysis by lunch type', *British Journal of Nutrition* (August 2010), 104(4): pp. 474–87.

3. Spence, S., Delve, J., Stamp, E., Matthews, J., White, M. and Adamson, A., 'Did school food and nutrient-based standards in England impact on 11–12Y olds' nutrient intake at lunchtime and in total diet? Repeat cross-sectional study', *PLoS One* (November 2014), 19, 9(11).

4. Zandian, M., Ioakimidis, I., Bergstrom, J., Brodin, U., Bergh, C., Leon, M., Shield, J. and Sodersten, P., 'Children eat their school lunch too quickly: an exploratory study of the effect on food intake', *BMC Public Health* (14 May 2012), 12: p. 351.

5. The American Academy of Pediatrics, 'Policy statement: the crucial role of recess in school', *Pediatrics* (January 2013), vol. 131, issue 1.

6. Parmer, S., Salisbury-Glennon, J., Shannon, D. and Struempler, B., 'School gardens: an experiential learning approach for a nutrition education program to increase fruit and vegetable knowledge, preference, and consumption among second-grade students', *Journal of Nutrition Education and Behaviour* (May–June 2009), 41(3): pp. 212–17.

7. DeCosta, P., Moller, P., Frost, M. and Olsen, A., 'Changing children's eating behaviour – a review of experimental research', *Appetite* (9 March 2017), 113: pp. 327–57.

8. Dannefer, R., Bryan, E., Osborne, A. and Sacks, R., 'Evaluation of the Farmers' Markets for Kids programme', *Public Health Nutrition* (December 2016), 19(18): pp. 3397–405.

9. Wiegand, S., 'Gender and obesity – what does "being fat" mean to boys and girls?', *Therapeutische Umschau* (June 2007), 64(6): pp. 319–24.

10. Bacchini, D., et al., 'Bullying and victimization in overweight and obese outpatient children and adolescents: An Italian multicentric study', *PLoS One* (25 November 2015), 10(11).

11. Jansen, P., et al., 'Teacher and peer reports of overweight and bullying among young primary school children', *Pediatrics* (September 2014), 134(3): pp. 473–80.

12. Olvera, N., Dempsey, A., Gonzalez, E. and Abrahamson, C., 'Weight-related teasing, emotional eating, and weight control behaviors in Hispanic and African American girls', *Eating Behaviour* (December 2013), 14(4): pp. 513–17.

13. Madowitz, J., Knatz, S., Maginot, T., Crow, S. and Boutelle, K., 'Teasing, depression and unhealthy weight control behaviour in obese children', *Pediatric Obesity* (December 2012), 7(6): 446–52.

14. Krukowski, R., West, D., Philyaw Perez, A., Bursac, Z., Phillips, M. and Raczynski, J., 'Overweight children, weight-based teasing and academic performance', *International Journal of Pediatric Obesity* (2009), 4(4): pp. 274–80.

15. Quick, V., McWilliams, R. and Byrd-Bredbenner, C., 'Fatty, fatty, two-by-four: weight-teasing history and disturbed eating in young adult women', *American Journal of Public Health* (March 2013), 103(3): pp. 508–15.

16. Lowes, J. and Tiggemann, M., 'Body dissatisfaction, dieting awareness and the impact of parental influence in young children', *British Journal of Health Psychology* (2003), vol. 8, issue 2, pp. 135–47.

17. Ackard, D. and Peterson, C., 'Association between puberty and disordered eating, body image, and other psychological variables', *International Journal of Eating Disorders* (March 2001), 29(2): pp. 187–94.

18. Slater, A. and Tiggemann, M., 'Little girls in a grown up world: exposure to sexualized media, internalization of sexualization messages, and body image in 6–9 year-old girls', *Body Image* (September 2016), 18: pp. 19–22.

19.	Garbett, K. and Diedrichs, P., 'Improving uptake and engagement with child body image interventions delivered to mothers: understanding mother and daughter preferences for intervention content', *Body Image* (2016), 19: pp. 24–7.

20.	Griffiths, C., Gately, P., Marchant, P. and Cooke, C., 'Cross-sectional comparisons of BMI and waist circumference in British children: mixed public health messages', *Obesity*, (2012), 20(6), pp. 1258–60.

21.	McDonald, S., Ginez, H., Vinturache, A. and Tough, S. (2016), 'Maternal perceptions of underweight and overweight for 6–8 years olds from a Canadian cohort: reporting weights, concerns and conversations with healthcare providers', *BMJ Open* (19 October 2016)m 6(10).

22.	Birch, L. and Davison, K., 'Family environmental factors influencing the developing behavioral controls of food intake and childhood overweight', *Pediatric Clinics of North America* (August 2001), 48(4): pp. 893–907.

23.	Carper, J., Orlet Fisher, J. and Birch, L., 'Young girls' emerging dietary restraint and disinhibition are related to parental control in child feeding', *Appetite* (2000), vol. 35, issue 2, pp. 121–9.

24.	Jansen, E., Mulkens, S. and Jansen, S., 'Do not eat the red food!: prohibition of snacks leads to their relatively higher consumption in children', *Appetite* (2007), vol. 49, issue 3, pp. 572–7.

25.	Butwicka, A., Lichtenstein, P., Frisen, L., Almqvist, C., Larsson, H. and Ludvigsson, J., 'Celiac disease is associated with childhood psychiatric disorders: a population-based study', *Journal of Pediatrics* (7 March 2017), epub ahead of print.

26.	Newens, K. and Walton, J., 'A review of sugar consumption from nationally representative dietary surveys across the world', *Journal of Human Nutrition and Dietetics* (April 2016), 29(2): pp. 225–40.

27.	Duyff, R., et al., 'Candy consumption patterns, effects on health, and behavioral strategies to promote moderation: summary report of a roundtable discussion', *Advances in Nutrition* (January 2015), 6(1): pp. 139S–46S.

Chapter 7

1.	McInnes, A. and Blackwell D., 'Self-reported perceptions of weight and eating behavior of school children in Sunderland, England', *Frontiers in Public Health* (14 February 2017), 5: p. 17.

2. Balantekin, J., Birch, L. and Savage, J., 'Family, friend, and media factors are associated with patterns of weight-control behavior among adolescent girls', *Eating and Weight Disorders*, 17 Mar 2017, epub ahead of print.

3. Neumark-Sztainer, D., Bauer, K., Friend, S., Hannan, P., Story, M. and Berge, J., 'Family weight talk and dieting: how much do they matter for body dissatisfaction and disordered eating behaviors in adolescent girls?', *Journal of Adolescent Health* (September 2010), 47(3): pp. 270–6.

4. Turner, P. and Lefevre, C., 'Instagram use is linked to increased symptoms of orthorexia nervosa', *Eating and Weight Disorders* (2017), epub ahead of print.

5. Stice, E., Gau, J., Rohde, P. and Shaw, H., 'Risk factors that predict future onset of each DSM-5 eating disorder: predictive specificity in high-risk adolescent females', *Journal of Abnormal Psychology* (January 2017), 126(1): pp. 38–51.

6. Haines, J., et al., 'Family functioning and quality of parent-adolescent relationship: cross-sectional associations with adolescent weight-related behaviors and weight status', *International Journal of Behavioural Nutrition* (14 June 2016), 13: p. 68.

7. Joseph, N., Nellivanil, M., Rai, S., Kotian, S., Ghosh, T. and Singh, M., 'Fast food consumption pattern and its association with overweight among high school boys in Mangalore City of southern India', *Journal of Clinical and Diagnostic Research* (May 2015), 9(5), pp. 13–17.

8. Sadler, R., Clark, A., Wilk, P., O'Connor, C. and Gilliland, J., 'Using GPS and activity tracking to reveal the influence of adolescents' food environment exposure on junk food purchasing', *Canadian Journal of Public Health* (9 June 2016), 107, suppl. 1: 5346.

9. Uribe, R. and Fuentes-Garcia, A., 'The effects of TV unhealthy food brand placement on children. Its separate and joint effect with advertising', *Appetite* (August 2015), 91: pp. 165–72.

10. Freeman, B., Kelly, B., Baur, L., Chapman, K., Chapman, S., Gill, T. and King, L., 'Digital junk: food and beverage marketing on Facebook', *American Journal of Public Health* (December 2014), 104(12), pp. 56–64.

11. Isasi, C., Ostrovsky, N. and Wills, T., 'The association of emotion regulation with lifestyle behaviors in inner-city adolescents', *Eating Behaviour* (December 2013), 14(4): 518.

12. Zandian, M., Ioakimidis, I., Bergstrom, J., Brodin, U., Bergh, C.,

Leon, M., Shield, J. and Sodersten, P., 'Children eat their school lunch too quickly: an exploratory study of the effect on food intake', *BMC Public Health*, 12 (2012): p. 351.

13.   Sawka, K., McCormack, G., Nettel-Aquirre, A. and Swanson, K., 'Associations between aspects of friendship networks and dietary behavior in youth: findings from a systematized review', *Eating Behaviour* (August 2015), 18: pp. 7–15.

14.   Dimitriou, D., Le Cornu Knight, F. and Milton, P., 'The role of environmental factors on sleep patterns and school performance in adolescents', *Frontiers in Psychology* (1 December 2015), 6: p. 1717; 'How much sleep do babies and kids need?', National Sleep Foundation, accessed online, 28 March 2017: https://sleepfoundation.org/excessivesleepiness/content/how-much-sleep-do-babies-and-kids-need.

15.   Buxton, O., Chang, A., Spilsbury, J., Bos, T., Emsellem, H. and Knutson, K., 'Sleep in the modern family: protective family routines for child and adolescent sleep', *Sleep Health* (1 May 2015), 1(1): pp. 15–27.

16.   Turel, O., Romashkin, A. and Morrison, K., 'A model linking video gaming, sleep quality, sweet drinks consumption and obesity among children and youth', *Clinical Obesity* (20 March 2017), epub ahead of print.

Index